Balancing in Heels

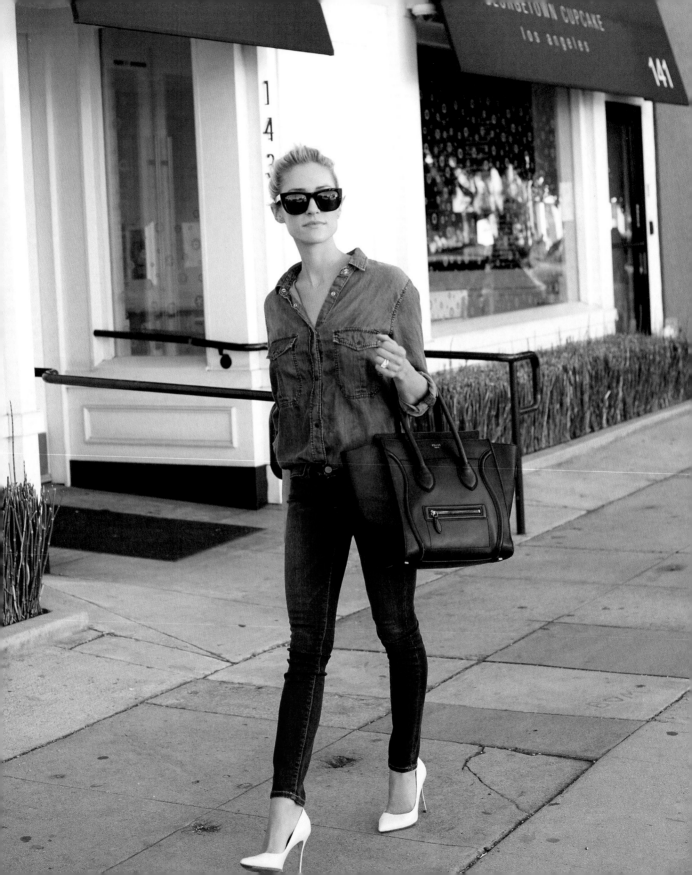

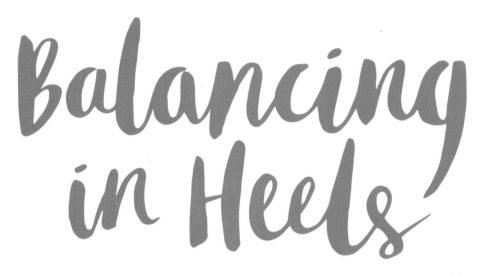

Balancing in Heels

My Journey to Health, Happiness, and Making It All Work

KRISTIN CAVALLARI

Photographs by Tec Petaja

RODALE.

RODALE
wellness

Live happy. Be healthy. Get inspired.

Sign up today to get exclusive access to our authors, exclusive bonuses,
and the most authoritative, useful, and cutting-edge information for health,
wellness, fitness, and living your life to the fullest.

Visit us online at RodaleWellness.com
Join us at RodaleWellness.com/Join

© 2016 by Kristin Cavallari
Photographs © 2016 by Tec Petaja

Rodale books may be purchased for business or promotional use or for special sales.
For information, please write to:
Special Markets Department, Rodale Inc., 733 Third Avenue, New York, NY 10017

Printed in the United States of America
Rodale Inc. makes every effort to use acid-free ♾, recycled paper ♻.

Photos from Kristin Cavallari's personal collection (pages 10, 16, 17, 23, 26, 29, 57 *except
bottom left*, 63, 64, 79 *bottom*, 139, 151, 167, 188, 192); Paul Archuleta/Getty Images (page 179 *top right*);
Jen Cooper (page 196); Gregg DeGuire/Getty Images (page 179 *top left*); Lilly Lawrence/Getty Images
(page 179 *bottom*); J. Merritt/Getty Images (page 57 *bottom left*); Amelia Moore Photography (pages 69,
70, 72); Sorella Muse/N. Anderson Studio (page 79 *top*); yonibunga/Shutterstock (page 25)

Book design by Rae Ann Spitzenberger
Hand lettering by The Lovely Drawer

Library of Congress Cataloging-in-Publication Data is on file with the publisher.
ISBN 978–1–62336–638–4   paperback

Distributed to the trade by Macmillan
2   4   6   8   10   9   7   5   3   paperback

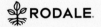

RODALE

Follow us @RodaleBooks on 🐦 📘 📌 📷

We inspire and enable people to improve their lives and the world around them.
rodalewellness.com

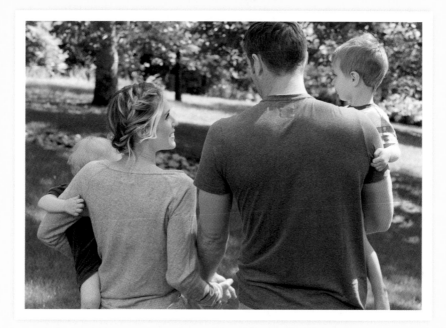

*For my babies, who inspire me to be
the best version of myself*

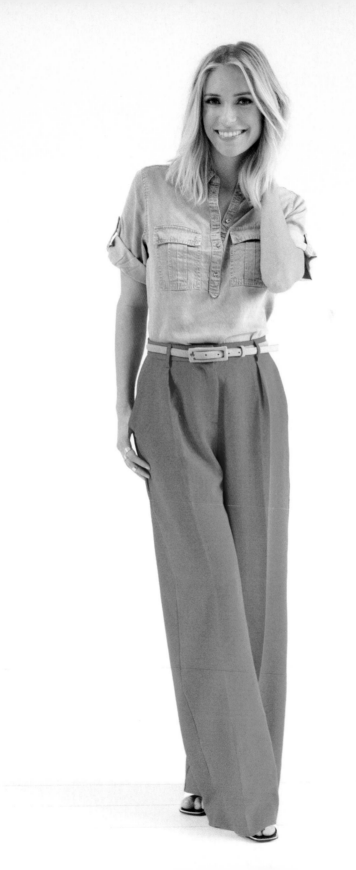

CONTENTS

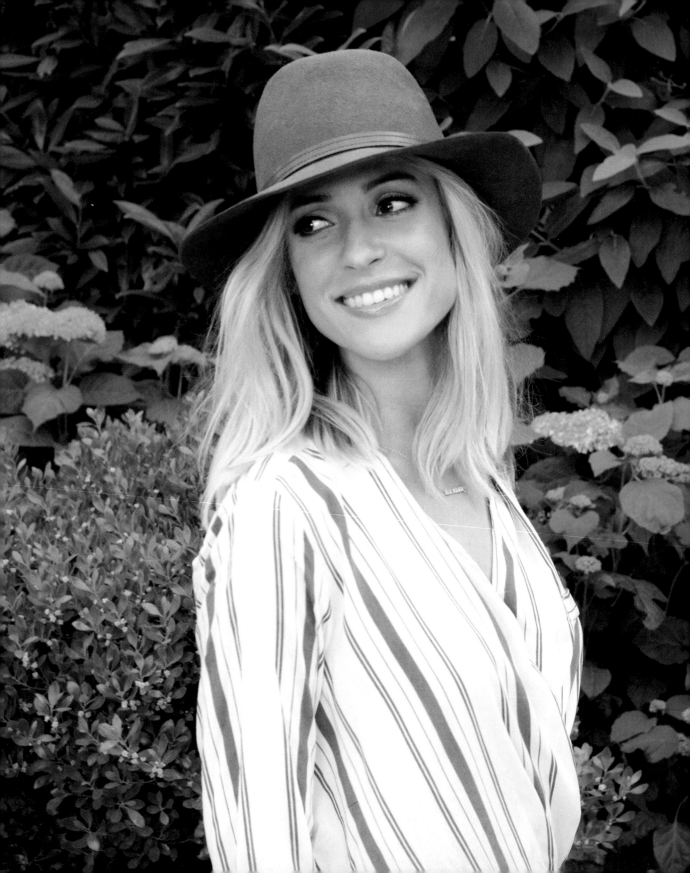

Introduction

IN MY JUNIOR YEAR OF HIGH SCHOOL, MTV SHOWED UP at my Laguna Beach, California, high school one January day and set up a booth in the quad. I was cast without even meeting the producers just because I was the link that tied everyone together. The show was titled *Laguna Beach: The Real Orange County,* and MTV started filming in 2004. It centered on the lives of five girls, including me, and three boys. Teenage drama began on the first episode and grew from there. The show was a wild ride—and an immediate hit.

Filming a super-successful reality television show when you are just 17 can do a number on your conception of reality. Like many teenagers, I had no self-awareness and thought only about myself, and that was amplified by starring on *Laguna Beach*, where I got professional accolades for being outspoken and wild. Being tough and rebellious felt like my real identity, and I thought I was in total control of my life. But it wasn't the whole picture. My relationships and the general ups and downs of that time and immediately after were often manipulated for dramatic effect by TV producers or even myself. Behind the scenes, I was uncomfortable and terrified of getting hurt. I often hung out with all the wrong people to avoid having to let anyone in. Plus, I never properly took care of myself, mentally or physically. The actual reality of that celebrity-filled, L.A.-industry–driven life was that I needed some serious growing up.

Remember, reality shows at this time were just starting to become popular—audiences *and* cast members know a lot more now than we did then. There was certainly a good deal to the show that wasn't "real," but as kids we got caught up in it anyway. It was easy to go along with made-up situations and not think much about the consequences. To keep things interesting, words were dubbed, scenes filmed months apart were shown in the same episode as though they were concurrent, and phone calls were faked (I would literally be on the phone with no one or sometimes

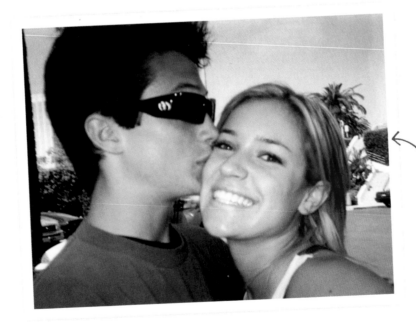

Good times with Stephen in my junior year of high school

with a producer). Pickup scenes were ordered and filmed in postproduction, when producers realized they needed something specific to keep their "story" going. I was a carefree, go-with-the-flow type of person, so I often didn't question things until it was too late . . . like the producers having me record "wild lines"—bits of audio to splice into whatever scene they wanted. If it wasn't a line I was completely comfortable with, they would tell me to just try it and they wouldn't use it if it didn't sound right. Ha, I soon learned my lesson about believing that!

Don't get me wrong, I wouldn't trade my experience on *Laguna Beach,* and later on *The Hills,* for the world. I had a blast filming the majority of the time and have beautiful footage of special moments with my friends, like prom and graduation. It was an experience that most people will never get, and I will always have a great story to tell. I loved the attention from the media (at 17 and 18, it was all new and exciting), but I struggled with people thinking I was someone I wasn't. Young girls all over the world were criticizing me for being a bitch, but media outlets loved it—that year was my biggest to date in terms of recognition and bookings for magazines and talk shows. Confusingly, the experience was the "making" of me professionally, but otherwise it was something I didn't feel had much to do with the real me. Though I was much more than the character they showed on TV, I still didn't even really know who I was.

> Though I was much more than the character they showed on TV, I still didn't even really know who I was.

GROWING UP

It wasn't until my early twenties that things changed. Once I left the reality shows, work—acting, hosting, fashion—became more meaningful. I began to surround myself with people whom I genuinely cared about, who in turn genuinely cared about me. After years in the public eye, I came to terms with my body and, most important, my true self. Finally, it wasn't until I had a child and got married, and in that order, that I realized how happy and centered I could be.

For the first time in my life, I know who I am. I'm pretty simple. I am a no-fuss, on-the-go kind of girl who knows exactly what she wants. I never settle. I always find a way to make things work, whatever those things are. I am a mother to two amazing little boys and a beautiful little girl, the wife of an NFL quarterback, and a girly girl who loves fashion and beauty. I'm a businesswoman who wears many hats (shoe and jewelry designer, TV host, and producer), a passionate health nut, and an enthusiastic home cook. I know my likes and dislikes. I understand what drives me. I know that I only want positive people in my life. In short, I've grown up and gotten my shit together. I've learned how to live a healthy, happy life.

That is not to say my life is perfect. I've been the lucky recipient of many great things, but I also have faced some tough times. Through all the trial and error of my adult life so far, I've changed a lot, and my priority is making good choices for my family and me. And I still have a lot to learn—I look forward to that. For example, over the years I've discovered that you cannot please everyone, no matter what you do. This is one of the best life lessons for surviving relationships and life in general. Let me repeat that: You cannot please everyone, no matter what you do. So I've stopped trying to please everyone and stopped living my life for other people. You have to do what makes *you* happy. When I was the wild teenager on *Laguna Beach,* I was hated for being a party animal. Now that I'm married and settled down, people say I'm boring. I can't win. So guess what? I don't concern myself with winning anyone over anymore. I live my life for me, not for how people want me to be.

LESSONS LEARNED

This book discusses my journey from reality stardom to real life—the good, the bad, and the ugly—explaining what truly makes me who I am and the lessons I learned along the way. The first two chapters include the biggest influences in my life, the people closest to me: my children and my husband. These sections are the most personal, showing how these people came into my life, how my identity has been shaped by them, and how I prioritize my future with them. After that, I dig into the topics I care about most, which have made me the healthiest and happiest I've ever been: the amazing effects of good food and exercise (including how my husband's type 1 diabetes has drastically improved through our diet), the joy of fashion and beauty, and the importance of my work. From the rules and choices I live by to the specifics of my recipes and workouts, I show what my life is all about. And throughout the book, I share the ways I balance it all. You have to figure out what your priorities are!

I don't expect this book to be a step-by-step guide for anyone else—I can't prescribe what will make another person healthy or happy—I only know what has worked for me. But I do hope that sharing my experiences in growing up and becoming a more independent, thoughtful woman will be helpful to others. I hope this book will encourage anyone who picks it up to go out there and get whatever it is she (or he!) wants in life. Happiness is a choice that we all have the ability to make, so choose wisely!

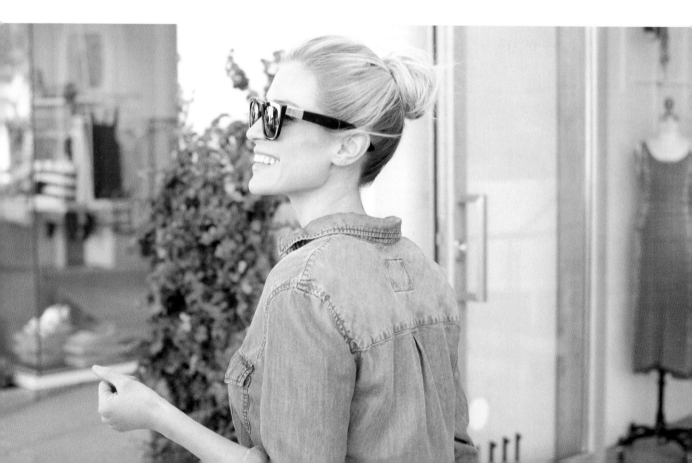

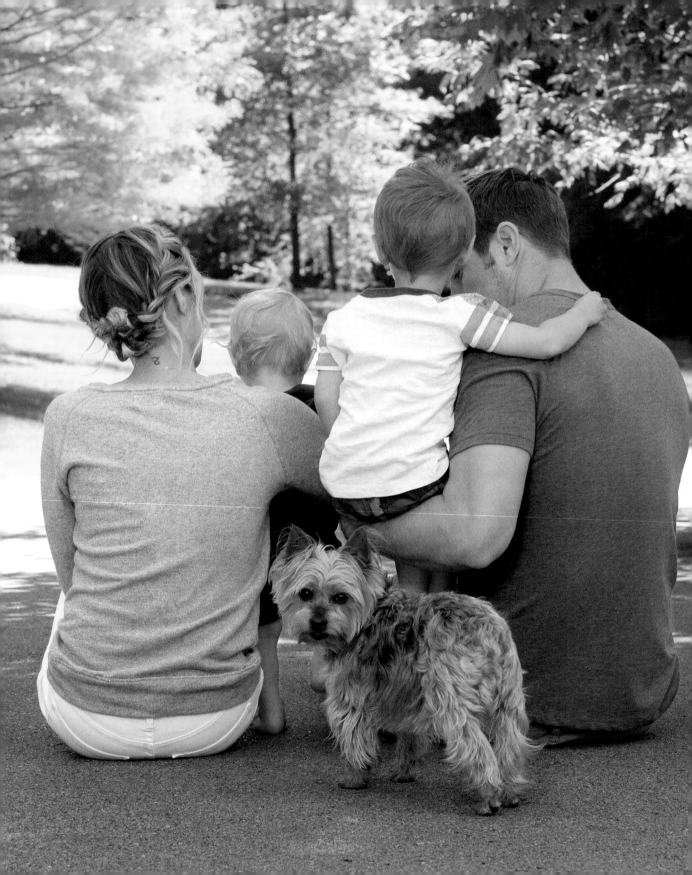

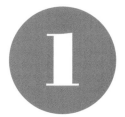

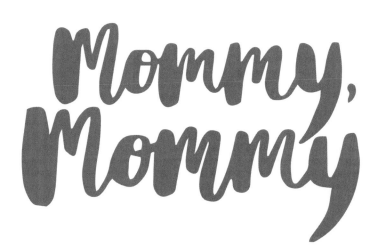

IF YOU HAD ASKED ME 10 YEARS AGO WHEN I WAS GOING TO HAVE kids, I would have told you I'd be the last one of my friends, because my entire world revolved only around me. At the time, I was more concerned about my career. Settling down was the last thing on my mind because I was having too much fun. But meeting Jay and a few years of growing up changed everything.

So, at just 24 years old, I became pregnant with my first. It was interesting timing considering Jay and I had only recently gotten back together after breaking off our engagement. But after 3 months of working on the relationship and being back together, we completely committed to our future together. Conceiving Camden was an in-the-moment decision that we both felt strongly about; it would end up being the best thing we ever did.

PREGNANCY

In November 2011, I had just finished taping the season finale of *Dancing with the Stars* and Jay was smack in the middle of the football season and had just broken his thumb. When I joined him in Vail where he was to get surgery on his hand, we took a pregnancy test, even though I thought it was a long shot since we hadn't been together much the previous month. Sure enough, the test showed up negative. Both of us felt surprisingly let down. But we carried on, spending Thanksgiving with my dad in Laguna Beach the following day. A couple of days later, we decided I should take another test because I was still unusually late. This

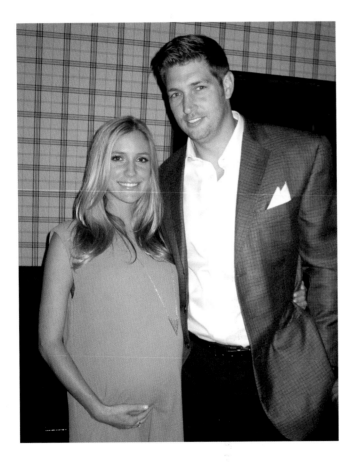

time the results were positive. We were both a little stunned, having convinced ourselves there wouldn't be a baby when the first pregnancy test had been negative. We kissed and hugged immediately and set off on this incredible journey together. It was an amazing time for us both. Being pregnant was the first time in my life where I felt like everything was on the right track and I was doing exactly what I was meant to be doing.

← Jay and I at an event for his charity, the Jay Cutler Foundation. I was 7 months pregnant with Camden.

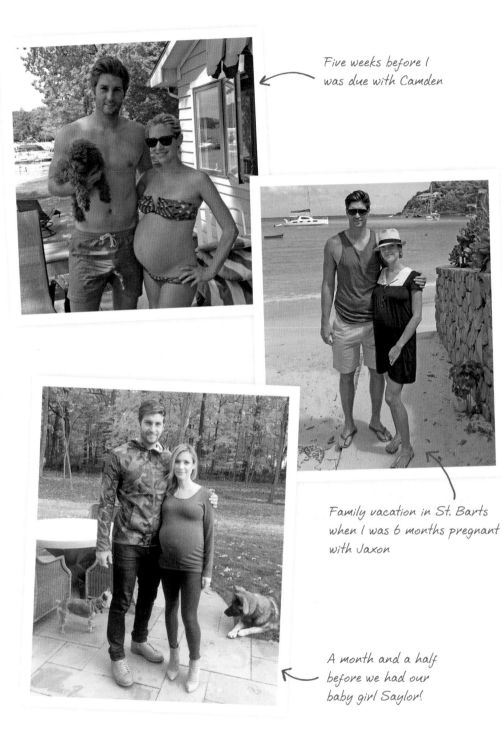

Five weeks before I
was due with Camden

Family vacation in St. Barts
when I was 6 months pregnant
with Jaxon

A month and a half
before we had our
baby girl Saylor!

FOOD

My eating was the number one thing that changed when I became pregnant—and that effect still resonates today. Becoming pregnant made me get serious about my health. Before pregnancy, I thought zero-calorie food was good for you and every calorie was equal. Deep down, I knew that my eating habits weren't truly healthful, but I put a lot of pressure on myself to be thin. I was my own worst critic: I hated the way I looked in certain pictures. Everyone around me was tiny, and I felt like I had to be too. I thought counting calories gave me control over my body.

> If it was good-quality, real food, I would give in to cravings and enjoy every second.

But when I became pregnant, I knew that everything I did, and especially what I ate, had a direct effect on my baby. I was solely responsible for the well-being of this little life and wanted only the best for him. That drastically changed my attitude toward food, which previously had been based only on eating a certain number of calories. For the first time in my life, I didn't care if I gained a lot of weight. It was a time to eat well and eat smart, and even to indulge in food that was forever off-limits in my prepregnancy life, including "fattening" things like cheese and pasta. I decided not to look at calories but instead to read ingredient labels and to reevaluate my ideas about avoiding so-called fattening foods. No matter what, I would eat only real food, no processed, chemical-laden junk. If it was good-quality, real food, I would give in to cravings and enjoy every second.

Pregnancy Snacks

I was constantly eating during pregnancy. I found it hard to eat big meals and loved grazing throughout the day. Eating smaller meals and snacking often cut down on my heartburn and kept my energy up. Some of my favorite snacks were:

- Hummus with carrot and celery sticks
- Guacamole with broccoli and cauliflower florets
- Homemade trail mix (nuts of choice, chocolate-covered goji berries, and dried cherries)
- Cheese slices with either an apple or flaxseed crackers
- A hard-cooked egg
- Smoothies (see the recipes on pages 20 and 21)

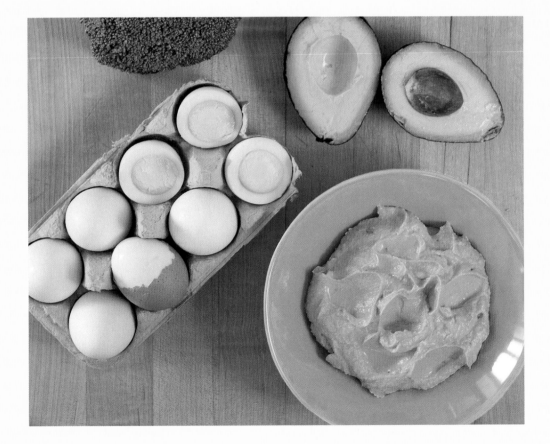

MINTY GREEN SMOOTHIE

I have a smoothie almost every morning, and this one is so good you will forget it's actually healthful. The peppermint in this smoothie saved me during the first trimester of my third pregnancy. I was incredibly nauseous, and this smoothie (which tastes like an ice-cream shake) calmed my stomach.

MAKES 1 SMOOTHIE

1¼ cups almond milk

1 avocado, peeled and pitted

1 handful spinach, stems removed

1 frozen banana

1 heaping tablespoon honey

¼ teaspoon spirulina powder

¼–½ teaspoon peppermint extract (not oil)

In a blender, combine the almond milk, avocado, spinach, banana, honey, spirulina, and peppermint extract to taste until smooth and creamy. Pour into a glass and enjoy.

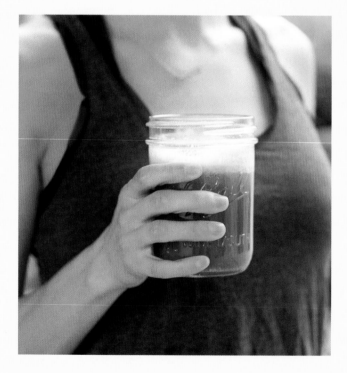

PEANUT BUTTER DELIGHT SMOOTHIE

MAKES 1 SMOOTHIE

1 cup almond milk

1 frozen banana

1 handful kale, stems removed

¼ cup peanut butter

1 tablespoon honey

1 scoop vanilla or plain protein powder

In a blender, combine the almond milk, coconut water, banana, kale, peanut butter, honey, and protein powder until smooth and creamy. Pour into a glass and enjoy.

CHOCOLATE FIX SMOOTHIE

MAKES 1 SMOOTHIE

1–1½ cups almond milk

½ avocado

1 handful spinach

1 frozen banana

1 heaping tablespoon raw honey

1 tablespoon raw cacao powder

1 teaspoon maca powder

In a blender, combine the almond milk, avocado, spinach, banana, honey, cacao, and maca powder until smooth and creamy. Pour into a glass and enjoy.

EXERCISING WITH THE BUMP

One of the most important things I did to take care of my body during pregnancy was work out. I didn't take it too hard and instead gave myself permission to slow down and go easy: I just wanted to move and get the blood flowing a few times a week. One of the main reasons I love working out is to keep myself sane. If I go longer than 5 days without doing something, I stress out easily and become irritable. Not good, especially with the added hormones and exhaustion of being pregnant. Exercise was important for my mental health as much as for the physical benefits.

Working out during my second pregnancy wasn't as easy, since my firstborn, Camden, was now on the scene. So the only thing I did was exercise at home (often while he napped) to DVD routines that mainly focused on my legs and butt. Sometimes Cam would hang with me while I followed the DVDs. To this day, he likes to "work out with Mommy" and kicks his legs and puts bands around his ankles like it shows on the DVDs. It's pretty darn cute.

WORKING OUT WHILE PREGNANT

Low-impact workouts a few times a week really helped my mind and my body while pregnant. Here are some of the exercises I loved.

- ▶ Walking uphill on the treadmill.
- ▶ Using a stairclimber—it's great cardio that isn't too hard on the body with the extra weight of a bump!
- ▶ Lifting light weights.

- ▶ Stretching with prenatal yoga—I loved this! It helped with the aches and pains in my lower back.
- ▶ Following DVDs of floor exercises— I did one called the Brazil Butt Lift, which obviously focused on my legs and butt.

TAKING CARE OF YOURSELF

I found all of my pregnancies to be relatively easy. I owe a huge part of this to diet but also to how I took care of myself physically. I learned how to listen to my body and to go easy when need be. If that meant I was in bed every night at 8:00 p.m., so be it! I also made an effort to be kind to myself in simple, everyday ways. Pampering myself at home on a Saturday required next to nothing and made me feel like a million bucks (see "Mini-Spa Day at Home" on page 25). And instead of meeting up with friends or leaving the house most nights, I simply savored coconut milk or cashew "ice cream" (see pages 227 and 228 for recipes) in bed and caught up on all my favorite shows (well, during the first pregnancy anyway!). It was heaven.

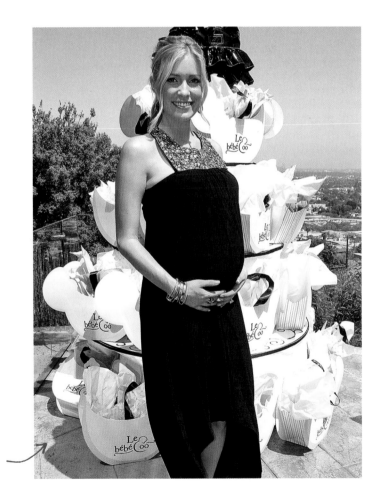

There is no better time to get in tune with your body than during pregnancy. It's an amazing thing to recognize exactly when you need to slow down. Truly knowing what you need and putting yourself first are often the best preventive medicine. I figured out how to read the signs pretty quickly and tried not to feel guilty or like I

My baby shower in L.A. when I was pregnant with Camden. Surrounded by all my best friends.

was missing out when I opted to stay home in pajamas instead of going to dinner with friends.

For example, I learned that attending a horse race in the summer is not the best activity for a pregnant woman. Who would have thought? But I hadn't had the foresight to realize that this sort of thing—which I'd always considered fun—was not going to work for me at 7 months pregnant. A group of us had decided to go to the Iroquois Steeplechase in Nashville (if you aren't familiar, it's like a smaller version of the Kentucky Derby), and I was optimistic that I could hang and enjoy myself without getting tired. But after an hour there—hot and surrounded by sweaty, drunk people—I knew I had made a mistake. Being the only sober person at a super-boozy event wasn't fun, plus I was physically uncomfortable just wandering around with everyone, with no place to sit. I wanted no part of it, so I decided to leave. Even though the after-party was held at our house, I was in bed early, perfectly content, while everyone partied the night away.

> Now, pregnant or not, I always try to get plenty of sleep.

I knew that if I had stayed and pushed myself, I would have been exhausted. And honestly, when I'm tired, I'm awful to be around. There's nothing I hate more than being grumpy and tired. I didn't always know this about myself, but it's one of the best things I figured out during pregnancy. Now, pregnant or not, I always try to get plenty of sleep.

Similarly, during my first pregnancy, I was traveling a lot for work and got pulled in every direction. I was back and forth to L.A. for shoe and jewelry design meetings. I was working on a pilot for a TV show that I was producing (unfortunately, the show never got picked up). I flew to New York City for paid events and had multiple photo shoots as well. It was too much. So I started saying yes only to jobs that I absolutely wanted to do. Being on planes while pregnant isn't my favorite thing. And overall, I was too tired and wanted to nest at home, so I had to be truly excited about whatever the offer was to accept. This prepared me for the time after having my babies, when I had to be even pickier about which jobs to take.

Mini-Spa Day at Home

A home spa day is an easy treat that you can give yourself, pregnant or not. I found it especially helpful in reconnecting with my body, which, during pregnancy, can often feel more like a vessel for a foreign object than a thing to be pampered. Here's what I do.

1. Enjoy a nice, long bath. You can add a few drops of lavender oil for a relaxing bath or a couple of drops each of peppermint and lemon oil for a pick-me-up. Rose oil is another girly option I love for its beautiful smell. It's also very sensual.

2. In the bathtub with the bathwater running, exfoliate your face with my "Homemade Coffee Face Scrub" (see the recipe on page 170). Then wipe off the scrub with a washcloth.

3. Apply a natural face mask (see my recipe for "Homemade Moisturizing Face Mask" on page 168). Leave it on for your time in the bath.

4. If your hair is dry, apply a coconut oil hydrating mask, then pull your hair back with a hair tie while the mask works its magic (see page 165 for specifics). Make sure to wash your hair before getting out of the tub. Coconut oil is great because one wash and it's gone.

5. After the bath, moisturize with body oil and whatever moisturizer you like for your face.

6. All the while, make sure to check yourself out in your bathroom mirror naked. The more time I spend with my naked self, the more I appreciate my body, especially while pregnant. A pregnant body is beautiful!

7. Give yourself a manicure and pedicure.

8. Finish the mini-spa with a blow-dry. For me, when my hair looks good, the rest doesn't matter.

SETTLING INTO PREGNANCY

Being pregnant gave me a newfound love and respect for my body that I didn't have before. It's a miracle that our bodies are capable of housing a baby for almost 10 months. If you don't feel great in your skin, just consider how spectacular our bodies are. We are able to give the gift of life! How amazing is that? When your belly is protruding so far you can't go 5 minutes without bumping into something, it will be hard to remember that this is a temporary situation (and one you will likely miss when it's gone—like I did!). But trust me, you will have your body back to yourself one day.

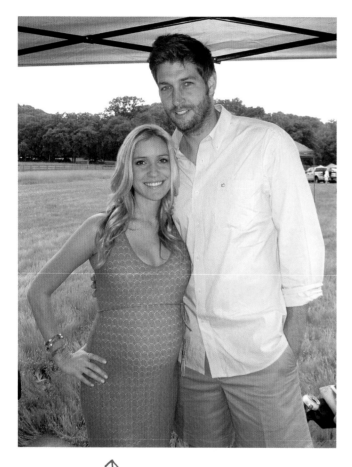

Seven months pregnant at Steeplechase

While I loved my pregnant body, especially my belly in the first few months, I started to get self-conscious toward the end. Many physical changes come along with being pregnant, and I found it hard to feel sexy. Besides the obviously expanding belly, my boobs got bigger (that was actually a plus), and I had a couple of pregnancy spots on my face from the sun and little bumps on the backs of my arms and thighs from hormones. Not always so pretty. With our bodies rapidly changing, it's no surprise that most of us need a little reassurance. As silly as it sounds, just telling yourself that you are beautiful is sometimes all you need. No matter how many times Jay told me I was beautiful, it didn't matter unless I felt good about myself. Being your own cheerleader can make all the difference. It all starts within ourselves!

But sometimes, of course, I needed outside reassurance too. I absolutely love Jay, but words are not his strong suit. Yes, I knew Jay loved me and still thought I was beautiful. I knew he wasn't going anywhere or looking at other women. But that didn't mean I didn't need to still hear occasionally that he thought I looked great. Also, I've noticed that guys are either totally turned on by pregnancy or a little freaked out by it. If your man falls more on the freaked-out scale, you aren't alone. Let's be honest: Having another human being growing inside you is pretty crazy, and it can be hard to express your own or your partner's trepidation without feeling ashamed. We can't assume our partners know what we are thinking and feeling. Once I discovered Jay was still getting comfortable with my body having an entire other human being living inside it, I realized he was going through his own changes as well. Knowing this made it easier to tell him how I was feeling. And once Jay knew all I needed to hear was that he thought I looked great, he made sure to say it often. Regarding self-image and comfort, the second and third pregnancies were much easier because of these conversations. Good communication is key!

> No matter how many times Jay told me I was beautiful, it didn't matter unless I felt good about myself.

I officially moved to Chicago when I was 6 months pregnant with Camden and couldn't wait to get everything organized. Jay and I moved into a new place and looked forward to starting a new life together. Getting the nursery ready and buying everything for Camden was surreal. I rode a roller coaster of emotions: I was excited but nervous to meet this little guy. I didn't know what to expect, and the unknown made me anxious. Remember that none of my friends had babies yet. I didn't have any exposure to a newborn, and I didn't know how I would handle the experience. There are so many stories about the first few months of motherhood being horrific, and that made me uneasy. I also valued my alone time and knew that would soon become a rarity.

Jay and I decided that staying connected was crucial during this period since I was still traveling a lot and he was working. We made regular date-night plans and tried to do as many fun things to prepare for Camden as possible, like hanging all the baby clothes up together and shopping for stuffed animals and bedding. Doing simple things like painting letters that spelled "Camden" was all part of the fun. As long as we were doing them together, it didn't matter how small or silly the tasks were, because this was a time in our lives we would always remember.

POSTBABY

Being a mom is truly the most natural thing I have ever done. I'm the most peaceful and happiest I've ever been, and am calm and confident most days. Of course, there were (and are!) plenty of day-to-day hiccups—like getting poop on myself and trying everything to get my darn baby to sleep(!)—but overall, with my kids, I finally feel like I have a real purpose.

> Being a mom is truly the most natural thing I have ever done.

With Camden, I was due in August, right in the middle of football training camp, when Jay lives in a college dorm for almost a month a few hours away from Chicago. So I was by myself the morning I went into labor, but I called Jay and he instantly hit the road. Since things didn't get serious for a couple of hours, he arrived home with enough time that we were able to go to the hospital together. Camden was born on August 8 after a relatively smooth 10-hour labor. Holding Camden for the first time was incredible; it was like nothing I had ever experienced. This kind of love was different. I had an instant need to protect and care for this little guy. And nothing else mattered in the world.

Luckily, Jay was able to stay with us the first 2 nights but then had to get back to work. He would be home in a couple of weeks, but then the football season would be kicking off. Bottom line, Jay wouldn't be around much for the next 5 months, so I would have to figure out how to survive on my own.

When our second child Jaxon was born, it was perfect. He arrived on May 7, during the time of year when Jay works only Monday through Thursday from 8:00 a.m. to noon. Having Jay around made a world of difference. I expected the second time to be harder, since I wouldn't be able to sleep when the baby slept (because Cam was around), but having Jay there to help out made the second newborn phase so much easier.

Our daughter, Saylor, was born November 23, a little more than halfway through the football season. Because of this timing, I was initially nervous about caring for a newborn with her two energetic brothers, but both our families live close by so I recruited my mom and mother-in-law for help. Camden was infatuated with Saylor from day 1 and helped as much as possible. Jaxon, on the other hand, took about a week to adjust to little Saylor being around, but once he did, he helped by bringing her toys and throwing diapers away for me.

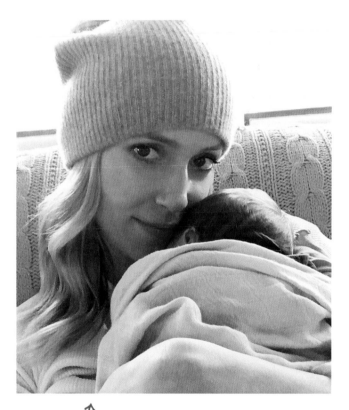

Newborn snuggles are the best! Days after being home with Saylor.

BREASTFEEDING AND SOLID FOOD

The food I give my children is one of the things I care most about. Just as I've learned over the years how important the food I feed myself is to my health and well-being, I know the same is even more true for my kids' development.

I realize how lucky I am that breastfeeding came easily to me. I had those babies latched on right away, and I am so thankful. Even though *that* part of breastfeeding was easy, the relentlessness of nursing a child was tough. Being tied down to the feeding schedule made getting anything done difficult, and it's obviously much harder to get sleep when you have to feed every couple of hours. Even though nursing was challenging at times, I committed to it since I know how beneficial breast milk is.

Breastfeeding Jaxon posed an extra challenge because he was sensitive to numerous foods, like eggs. Eggs are in just about everything! It took awhile

Easy, Healthy Snacks to Eat While Breastfeeding

Every mom has her own concerns about what to eat when breastfeeding. Here are some things I loved to eat between meals since I was hungry *all the time.*

- ▶ Organic apple with raw almond butter (Don't be skimpy with the almond butter—I would eat up to ½ cup at a time.)

- ▶ Grass-fed meat bar (similar to beef jerky; I especially like Epic brand, which comes in a few different flavors.)

- ▶ Quesadilla made with raw goat's milk Cheddar cheese and sprouted tortillas (I ate these until I realized my babies were sensitive to dairy.)

- ▶ Homemade trail mix with nuts of choice (I use walnuts, almonds, and cashews), chocolate-covered goji berries, and dried cherries

- ▶ Smoothie (I love protein smoothies made with protein powder, almond milk, berries, and spinach for extra iron.)

Dark leafy greens help promote milk flow while breastfeeding.

to figure out exactly what he couldn't tolerate—pinpointing allergens with an elimination diet doesn't happen overnight. And Jax was often uncomfortable due to itchy skin from eczema. It was pretty stressful. Anyone with a fussy baby can attest to that!

The more I talked to other moms about what I was going through, the more I realized many women aren't aware that a percentage of what you eat goes straight to your baby via breast milk. That's why a good diet is so important. Your little one is relying on you for good nutrition. (See Chapter 3 for more details on diet.) While breastfeeding, I tended to eat more protein and made sure I constantly ate tons of dark, leafy greens. I also drank a ridiculous amount of water and no other liquids. Sadly, I couldn't eat dairy or onions, because they made both boys fussy. And again, with Jax, I couldn't eat most store-bought foods because of his egg allergy. *That* was difficult.

Once I stopped breastfeeding each kid and we ran out of my stock of frozen breast milk, we put them on a homemade goat's milk formula (both grew out of their dairy sensitivity by then). I'm not a fan of soy (it's usually genetically modified; more about that later), and both Cam and Jax have sensitivities to cow's milk—and unfortunately, soy and cow's milk are the only two options for store-bought formula available right now. Goat's milk is the closest thing out there to human breast milk. Plus, it is more easily digested than cow's or soy milk. Giving goat's milk to children is popular in Europe and other parts of the world. Goat's milk itself is not enough, though, so Jay and I, along with our pediatrician, came up with a formula recipe for our kids, which I now share with you.

As a mother, I would rather feed my baby these real, organic ingredients than a heavily processed store-bought formula that contains "glucose syrup solids," which is another name for corn syrup solids, maltodextrin, carrageenan, and palm oil. Even organic formulas contain these controversial ingredients. In our homemade formula, cod-liver oil provides all the DHA and vitamin D your little one needs, and blackstrap molasses contributes vitamins and minerals like iron and calcium (though you might need to supplement with a little more blackstrap molasses should your child experience constipation). Coconut oil is one of nature's greatest fat sources, and olive oil is another healthy fat. The main component of breast milk is carbohydrates, which is why maple syrup comes into our recipe. While I wholeheartedly believe in this formula, it's important to talk to your pediatrician first before feeding it to your little ones.

> As a mother, I would rather feed my baby these real, organic ingredients than a heavily processed store-bought formula.

GOAT'S MILK FORMULA

FILLS FOUR 8-OUNCE BOTTLES, FOR BABIES UP TO 1 YEAR OLD*

Formula Base

4 cups (32 ounces) filtered water

¼ cup goat's milk powder (we like CapraMilk)

¼ cup pure organic maple syrup

2½ teaspoons good-quality extra virgin olive oil

¼ teaspoon unflavored cod-liver oil

¼ teaspoon unsulfured blackstrap molasses

For Each Bottle

1 teaspoon coconut oil

Probiotics (see Note)

1 **To make the formula base:** In a medium saucepan, gently warm the water, milk powder, maple syrup, olive oil, cod-liver oil, and molasses over medium heat, whisking to ensure that there are no clumps of milk powder. When everything is warmed and thoroughly combined, fill four 8-ounce bottles. Store in the refrigerator until ready to use, or for up to 1 day.

2 **To prepare a bottle for feeding:** Warm the formula and add the coconut oil and probiotics, shaking well to combine.

3 If your baby gets constipated, add more blackstrap molasses, ⅛ teaspoon more per batch. Once your baby is better, you can back off a little.

Note: I give my children ½ teaspoon of probiotics per day, split between their total number of bottles. Talk with your pediatrician about what is right for your kids.

*Once your baby is 1 year old, use ½ cup goat's milk powder instead of ¼ cup to make a richer formula.

POSTBREASTFEEDING

I'm equally concerned about my kids having nutritious meals and real food. My kids eat the same as I do: real, whole food. I'm not so super-strict that they can't have sweets at all or sample whatever they want at a birthday party, but when we're home, there's no processed food.

Camden loves to cook with me. Eating real food means we need to cook a lot, so I'm glad he's interested in the process. He doesn't actually help much, but he keeps me company by sitting on the counter and playing with the utensils. His favorite thing to make is "muffys," or muffins. He does help with those by putting the paper liners in the pan. When I'm burnt out and not wanting to cook, Jay picks up my slack. It's nice because he is pretty good in the kitchen as well!

Dinnertime is very important. The kids eat whatever Jay and I eat, and we all sit down at the dinner table without the distraction of TV or phones. I grew up like that, and I want to maintain these family-focused meals with my kids: I think it's crucial to connect and talk during dinner.

DIP IT

Kids love dipping foods into sauces, be it ranch dressing or barbecue sauce or the ubiquitous ketchup (not a vegetable in my book, but still okay!). Some of these sauces you can make yourself (see the Ranch Dressing recipe on page 219), but sometimes the convenience of store-bought is hard to beat. When buying condiments for kids:

- Read the ingredient label and strive to avoid high fructose corn syrup and other scary or controversial ingredients (see Chemicals in Surprising Places on page 91).

- Go for an option that has the fewest ingredients.

- Buy organic when possible.

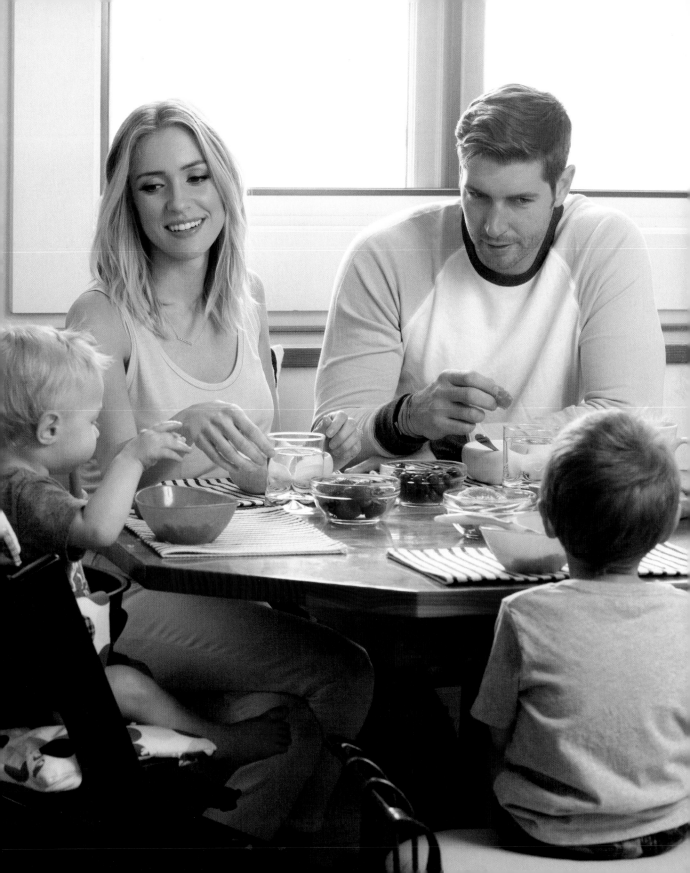

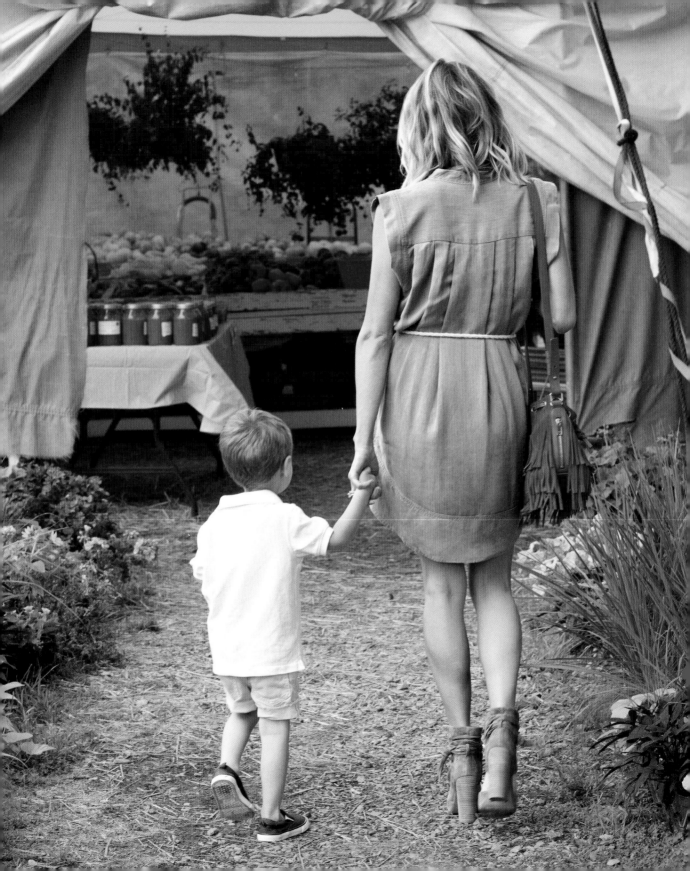

Like all children, mine go through phases of not wanting to eat very much or being unwilling to eat certain things. Camden is pretty easy to convince by giving him either homemade ranch dressing or store-bought organic ketchup (see "Dip It" on page 34) to dip his food in. The kid loves some dip! Another trick is to sneak greens into smoothies and muffins (see pages 20–21 and 205 for the recipes), since the taste of the greens vanishes in those foods. But overall, I believe that if youngsters start out eating well and are involved in the food-preparation process, they are pretty willing to keep trying new things. Since my kids don't have much processed food, they can't want what they've never had!

Dinners That Kids Love

- Healthy mac and cheese with brown rice pasta, grated raw goat's milk Cheddar, some grass-fed butter, and cooked broccoli thrown in for a green
- Mom's Peanut Butter Chicken (See the recipe on page 207.)
- Eggplant Parmesan made with buffalo mozzarella
- Homemade pizza with store-bought dough (we buy frozen gluten-free dough), buffalo mozzarella, and tons of veggies (My boys like spinach and red peppers.)
- Lettuce cups with ground chicken meat, carrots, and hoisin sauce (I like to make my own sauce.)

EXERCISING POSTBABY

Getting back in shape after the baby can be tough. It's a strange thing to look in the mirror and still look 5 months' pregnant even though the baby is by your side. And can we talk about how bizarre your belly feels? Like Jell-O! I've never had anything even *close* to a six-pack, but pressing on a stomach that jiggles like a bowl of mush was not something I was accustomed to.

To be honest, I didn't have a terribly hard time losing my baby weight. With my first two pregnancies, I gained 25 pounds, which for my body weight and height was exactly how much I was supposed to gain. The first 15 pounds fell off within the first couple of weeks, but the other 10 were a bit more stubborn.

I started working out after about 4 weeks with both Camden and Jax. I began slowly, sometimes only walking for 30 minutes with the baby in the stroller. I loved workout DVDs because they were easy to follow at home. I keep light weights at home as well. It wasn't long before another 5 pounds fell off, but the little pooch took a bit longer to finally say goodbye. Breastfeeding helped massively. I was hungrier breastfeeding than I was when I was pregnant. Your body burns a ton of calories when you breastfeed, and it's important to eat a lot so your body has the energy to produce milk.

Easy Ways to Get Back in Shape with Baby

- Exercise to workout DVDs at home during nap time or while your baby plays.

- Go for walks around the neighborhood with your baby in the stroller.

- Give baby to your hubby and take a nice trip to the gym!

- Run the stairs in your house and/or do lunges around the family room. Situps with baby work great too.

BEING KIND TO YOURSELF

My ego was too big to hire any help when I had Camden. I thought people expected me to ask for help or engage a nanny, and I was determined to prove them wrong. Also, I wanted to prove to myself that I could do it. When Jay had to work, I had my mom come with me and Cam when I traveled for work, but that was it. But after Cam, I learned that it's okay to accept help when offered (even to seek it sometimes!), to not try to do everything, and to let certain things go. Even during the most challenging moments of raising my kids, I still know I'm exactly where I'm meant to be.

To be honest, I was a zombie when Camden was first born, and in retrospect, I went back to work a little too soon. When he was 7 weeks old, I flew to Los Angeles with him for three back-to-back photo shoots and then took the red-eye to New

TAKING CARE OF YOU AFTER YOU'VE JUST HAD A BABY

▶ If friends and family offer help, accept it! I don't like people doing things for me, but having my mom take out the trash and make dinner once in a while made life with a new baby so much easier.

▶ Find a hobby or activity that you can fit into your busy schedule—cooking, crocheting, and reading are all great ideas. Even organizing—I will literally organize anything . . . there's nothing I love more! Learning or doing something new was helpful to making me feel like my life was not entirely about the baby.

▶ Don't worry about the baby weight. Just focus on the miracle that your body went through and know the weight will come off with time.

▶ You've heard it a million times, but get as much sleep as you can. Sleep when the baby sleeps.

▶ Don't stress about the small stuff. So dishes are piling up in the sink—who cares? You will get to them eventually. For now, just focus on sleep.

York City for more work before returning home to Chicago. Luckily, my mom came with me, but even still, I was constantly breastfeeding and getting up through the night, and I absolutely burned the candle at both ends.

So I started to say yes only to jobs that truly excited me. If it didn't fit into my brand or if it took me out of town for too long, I skipped it. After Camden was born, I received a ridiculously inflated six-figure offer to do a bikini photo shoot and say I lost my baby weight by taking a certain diet pill. I won't lie to you, that amount of money was tempting! But doing the shoot would go against everything I believe in, so I passed. The amazing thing about being pickier about which jobs to take is that I think it's made my work better. While I certainly work less, and I'm very lucky to be able to be selective (that's not a reality everyone lives, I know!), I also feel like I am working smarter. Because there is a self-imposed limit on the work I will take on, I choose the best things: projects that inspire me the most and fit the best within my brand. That makes the time I spend away from my family valuable and powerful—and I am a better mom and wife because of these creative outlets.

> I started to say yes only to jobs that truly excited me.

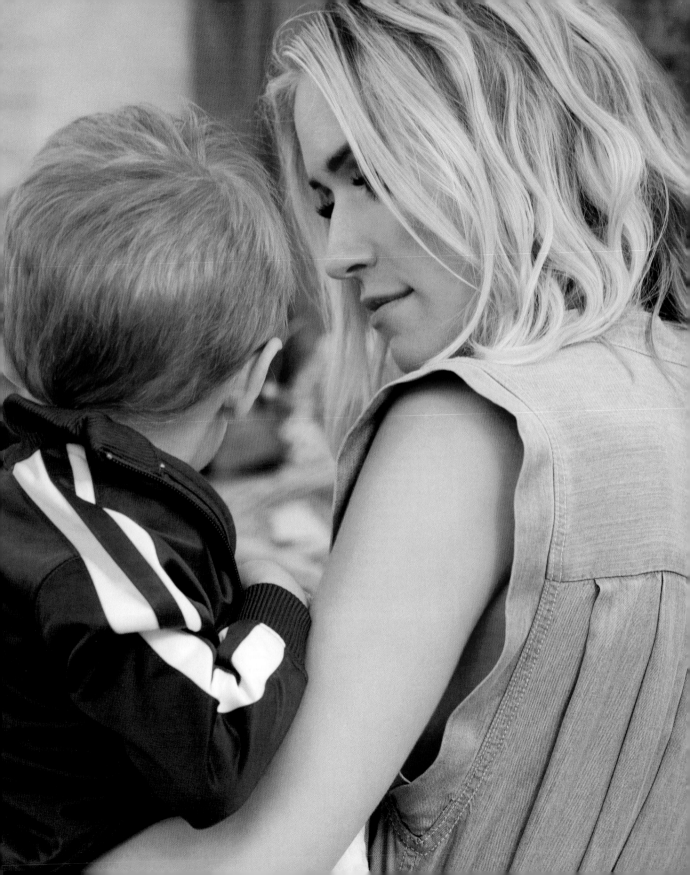

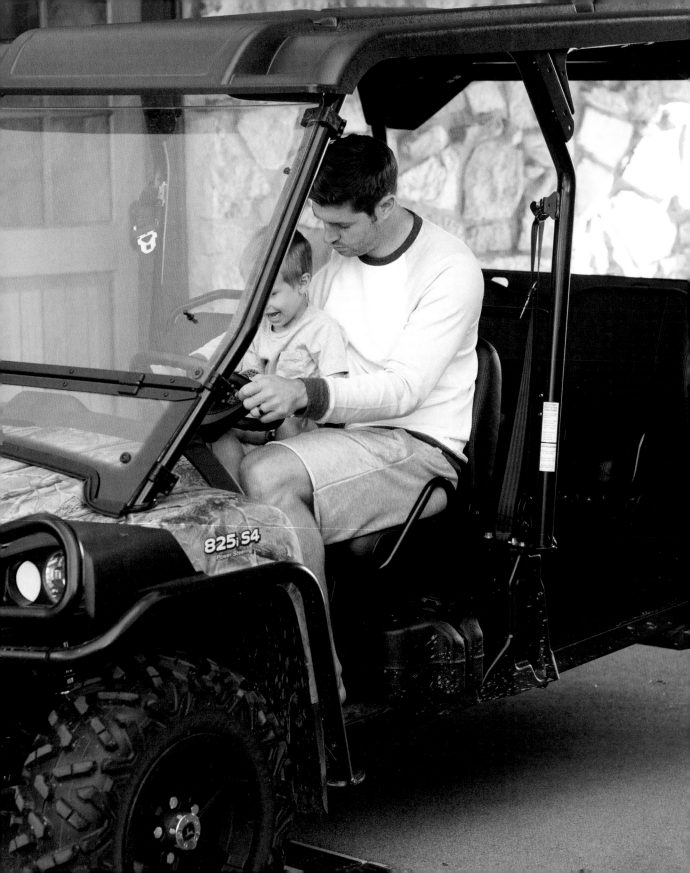

PARENTING WITH A PARTNER

I always knew Jay would be a good dad. He actually wanted kids when I met him, whereas I thought I wasn't quite ready yet. He wanted a big family and couldn't wait to get going.

Seeing your partner as a great father is the best feeling in the world. When a man is involved and changes diapers without being asked, you know you've found a good one. That's Jay. He's been hands-on since day 1 and didn't think twice about it. That's been incredibly attractive. I love seeing the man I love, love being a father.

As sexy as it is to see Jay as an amazing dad, it doesn't mean he and I don't still have our ridiculous fights about the kids! When everyone is sleep deprived and on edge, little ones' constant needs can put a strain on a relationship. As always, you have to work hard at achieving a great working relationship, especially with new babies in the house. Luckily, Jay and I had a solid foundation and some good tools to use (thanks to our therapist—see below) when things got stressful.

When you have kids, even if you are able to set aside the time to really talk to your partner, sometimes all you end up discussing is diapers and breastfeeding. Playing a game with your partner can change it up and open the door to talking about more interesting things! Jay and I play our version of 20 questions (not the

::

STAYING CONNECTED WITH YOUR PARTNER

It's tough to find quality time with your partner when you have young kids. Here are some things Jay and I did when we needed to reconnect.

▶ Though it's usually the last thing you want to do, ask a family member or good friend to watch the baby for an hour so just the two of you can get out of the house. Grab a casual dinner and simply talk.

▶ Put the baby in the stroller and go for a walk together.

▶ Eat dinner together after baby has gone to sleep. Even if you are just making scrambled eggs or ordering in Thai, light candles!

version for the car). Ask each other 20 random personal questions, things as small as "Diet Coke or Pepsi?" or "Favorite movie?" (even if you already know the answer) or as big as "What's your favorite memory from growing up?" or "What are you most thankful for right now?" or "What's the biggest lesson you've learned this year?"

The second time around was harder for me because I was spending the bulk of the time with Jaxon, the new baby. When you're breastfeeding, that's naturally going to be the case. I wanted Jay to take baby Jax when I wasn't breastfeeding so that I could hang with Cam, but that plan didn't always happen. And I would get frustrated in the middle of the night when I would be awake breastfeeding while watching Jay sleep soundly beside me. Being the mom of an infant often means most of the work falls on us, so it's easy to get upset, even though there isn't much we can do. Physically (and emotionally) we go through quite a bit in those early months. It's all part of the job. Once I started pumping and storing up a ton of milk, I was able to drop one breastfeeding at night and instead have Jay do a feeding with a bottle. That helped me a lot—not only could I sleep more but Jay could carry some of the load and have bonding time with his child. These lessons have come in handy with baby number three.

Tips for New Dads

- ▶ Make dinner. It doesn't have to be fancy—it's the thought that counts!

- ▶ Wash the bottles and breast pump parts—it's an endless job, and your partner will thank you every time! There is nothing worse to a mom than needing to pump and facing a sinkful of dirty nozzles and bottles.

- ▶ Change the baby's diaper after night feedings so your partner can go back to sleep.

- ▶ Offer to take a night feeding (if you use formula or there is enough pumped breast milk saved up).

- ▶ Write your partner a letter just saying she's doing an amazing job. Letting her know you appreciate everything she's doing goes far!

SETTLING INTO PARENTHOOD

Certain things had to fall by the wayside when I became a parent. In the early months, I went days without washing my hair and wore the same yoga pants until they started to smell. On days I was alone, I wouldn't brush my teeth sometimes until Camden took his first nap. Who am I kidding? That sometimes *still* happens when I'm alone with the kids! While I'm not exactly proud of these moments, I do realize that "letting go" is another way of prioritizing our family's overall happiness over the day-to-day mess. In that regard, I am happy to be a bum for a day or two!

Keep in mind that I am one of the most organized and type A people you will meet; everything has its spot, and I know if one little thing has been moved. After I had kids, I had to release some of those type A urges or I would have driven myself crazy. I didn't envision my life with toys sprawled across the living room floor. There are ways to make it more manageable (see "How to Deal with Kids When You Are Super Type A" on page 47), but the bottom line is, my house definitely looks different with kids around! Accepting that change has been freeing and made my life less stressful.

> After I had kids, I had to release some of those type A urges or I would have driven myself crazy.

But for all the exhaustion and hands-on time with an infant, I also realized something else with Cam, my first baby. Newborn babies sleep ALL. THE. TIME. Plus, Jay was away at work the majority of the time, and I was in a new city with only a couple of familiar faces. So I needed something to do at home that still felt productive and that I could do whenever. I'd always wanted to learn to cook, so one day I simply decided to start. I googled recipes and bought a couple of cookbooks. At the time, the most I could do was boil an egg! I found cooking to be therapeutic and a nice break from reality. I stumbled upon yet another new love in my life: I had Cam and I had cooking. So what if I was in the same dirty yoga pants? I was a happy girl.

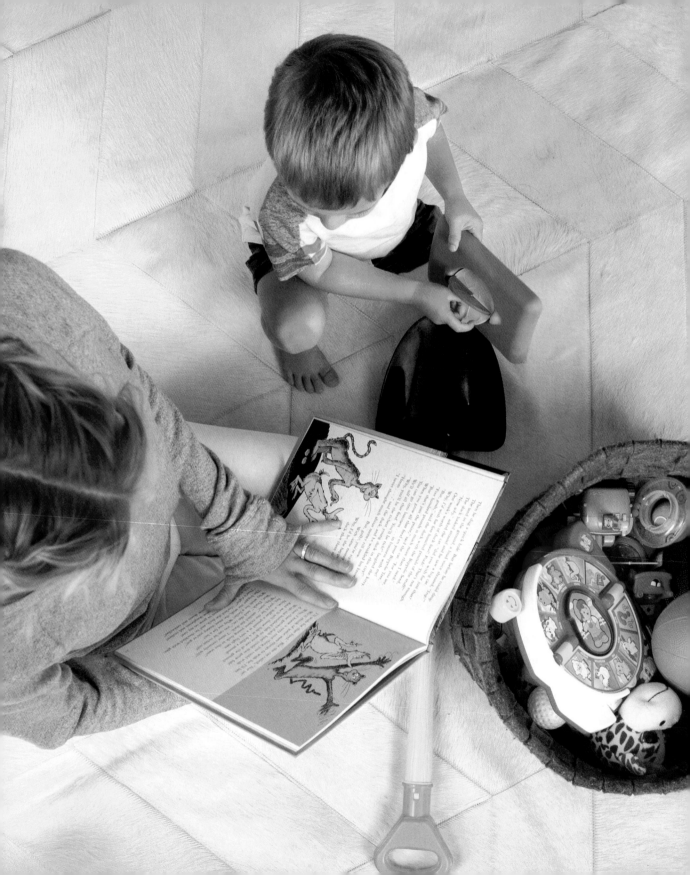

When it's just you and the baby at home, you have a tendency to get wrapped up in that focus. The entire world becomes the baby, and for me that isn't necessarily healthy. The power of friends quickly became apparent. When I first moved to Chicago, I had only one good friend nearby, and she was nowhere near settling down. She was out having fun almost every night while I had spit-up on all my clothes and could barely find time to brush my hair. Even though we were in two different orbits, that friendship was and still is so important. She gives me the occasional opportunity to escape my baby world, even for an hour at lunch. She reminds me of who I am, beyond a mom, and makes me laugh when she tells tales of her adventures. Just because she doesn't have kids doesn't mean we still don't enjoy each other and have a lot in common. Becoming a mom doesn't mean we have to lose ourselves. I'm not the kind of girl to let being a mom define me. Yes, it's a huge part of who I am, but it's not *me*.

Similarly, when Camden was a newborn, I brought him to Los Angeles with me for work. I decided to leave him with my mom for a couple of hours and squeezed in dinner with some friends. I could have argued that I already had too much going

HOW TO DEAL WITH KIDS WHEN YOU ARE SUPER TYPE A

▶ Create hiding spots for the toys in the rooms that the kids play in: a cupboard in the living room, for example. The more places you have to house all of their coloring books, balls, etc., the less of it you'll see!

▶ Dedicate one section/drawer/cabinet in the kitchen just for their stuff (sippy cups, plates, bowls, etc.).

▶ Make it a habit to have the kids pick up their own toys before nap time and bedtime. They love the praise they get after picking everything up, and it makes them more willing to help out.

▶ Try to make peace with the occasional mess. Simply accept that STUFF is going to be around! I only pick up at the end of the day so I'm not constantly cleaning.

on (and I did!). And friends were the last thing on my mind in the flurry of my baby's minute-to-minute needs. But here's the point: That friend time was the most important thing I did during that busy trip to L.A. Even though I could barely keep my eyes open before I showed up for the dinner, once there with my friends, I was reenergized. I felt a million times better after I took some time for myself and my needs. In short, if you can see your friends occasionally, even for a brief visit, it is one thing that is worth *not* sleeping for.

MINI FRIEND DATES

WITH THE BABY

▸ Put the baby in the stroller and go to the park. I found it nice to be around other moms with their kids while getting fresh air.

▸ Go to brunch/lunch (especially when the baby is napping, since newborns can sleep through just about anything!).

▸ Host brunch/lunch at your home and have your friends bring food.

▸ Take a baby class with another friend. It's a way to meet other moms, and the babies love the classes.

WITHOUT THE BABY

▸ Take a workout class together.

▸ Get manicures and pedicures.

▸ Go to a nice dinner and get dressed up—you should even have a glass of wine!

▸ Go to a friend's house, order in, and watch trash TV. The ultimate girl time!

Traveling with a Baby

Camden was a pro traveler by the time he was a year old. He was never a problem on flights, and I never worried too much about him. Then during one trip from Chicago to L.A., he happened to be teething. He managed to be a good sport, and he was content watching shows on the iPad, since he didn't typically get to do that. But as we were landing, he started screaming and crying for no apparent reason. Everyone around me was giving me dirty looks, but nothing I did would make Cam stop. Next thing I knew, he had projectile vomited all over himself and me. Then he did it again. Then again. Then *again.* Four times! Vomit everywhere. Poor Cam was crying hysterically, and I was mortified when the crew came by and tried to clean up. Plus, I didn't have a change of clothes for either of us, and we smelled awful. Lesson learned: When traveling with kids, always be prepared. Be sure to carry on:

- A change of clothes for both of you (because projectile vomit, or the like, can happen)

- Snacks (I bring a whole variety so that I have whatever they're in the mood for.)

- Bottles/sippy cups (I bring more than enough because my kids would drink a thousand sippy cups of coconut water and milk a day. Beverages are a great distraction.)

- An iPad (Normally, I don't let the kids watch screens more than 15 to 20 minutes a day, but anything goes on a flight! I download all kinds of shows and games that they like. Anything Mickey Mouse is a hit.)

- Suction-cup toys (great to stick onto the tray table)

One more tip for traveling with baby: Don't stress too much. Your baby will pick up on your anxiety and start stressing out too. Remember, many people have been there, so know that deep down—even if they are frustrated with the noise—your fellow travelers are probably sympathetic!

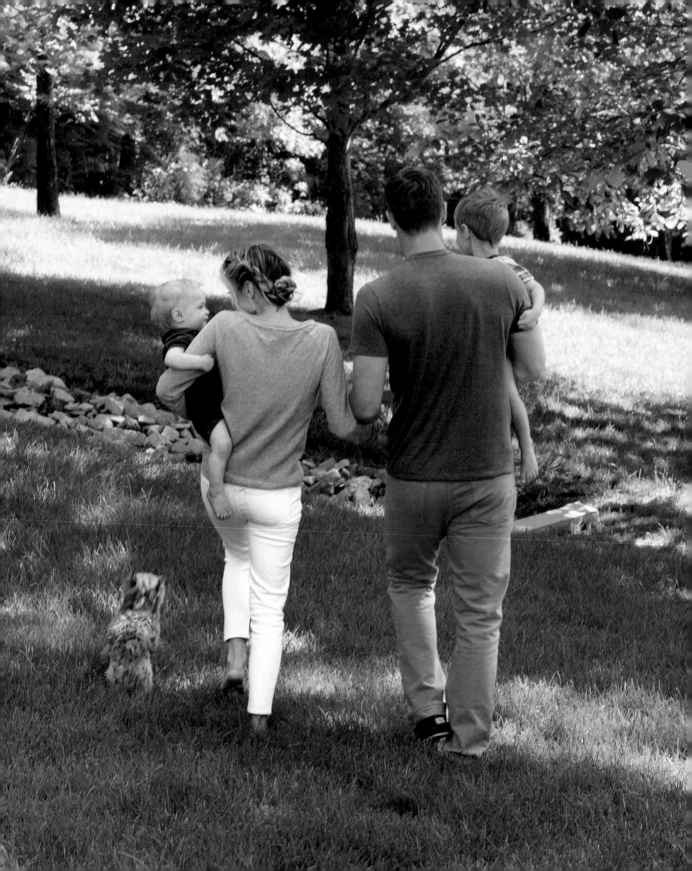

MOMMY OF TWO (OR THREE!)

I found baby number two to be much easier all around, especially when it came to knowing what to do and what to expect with labor and delivery. Plus, Jay was actually around this time since Jax was born during the football off-season!

We approach any potential sibling rivalry head-on. My biggest concern before we brought Jax home was how Camden was going to take it. I didn't want him to be upset or feel replaced. We decided to move Camden into his big-boy room before Jax was on the scene, so we had time to get him as excited as possible with his toddler bed and with decorating his new room in a sports theme. (He truly does love sports, not just because of Jay.) We also bought presents for Camden to bring home with us from the hospital. We pretended they were from Jaxon; while a bit deceptive, this strategy worked like a charm and created some immediate brotherly love! We did the same with Jax when the new baby came home. We often tell Camden and Jax what good brothers they are—that helps too.

The only thing that isn't easier with more than one kid is there's no downtime. Before baby two, one parent could watch the baby while the other took a shower or got dinner ready, but now it's man on man, or worse! The only moments you have to yourself are during nap times. This is why getting little ones on the same nap schedule is crucial! As they switch from three to two and two to one naps, they will probably be off for a few months, but once they're both taking one nap those few hours of downtime are heaven.

Balancing It All

For me to be happy, I need two things in my life: work and family. Once I had kids, I put them first, no matter what. My family is my number one priority, and nothing can change that. But I am very lucky to be able to be a full-time mom the majority of the time while still working on projects that excite and energize me. I say yes only to things I absolutely love and want to do and that fit into my schedule. While that limits my work (one could even say my work "suffers" for it), I tend to see my selectiveness as a positive, since the work I choose is the most fulfilling for me and keeps my priorities straight. While I wouldn't say I have it all, I do have what I want the *most*. I'm able to keep my creative juices flowing and to call fashion "work" while maintaining a normal, fulfilling family life where I can be home with my kids and make them dinner most nights.

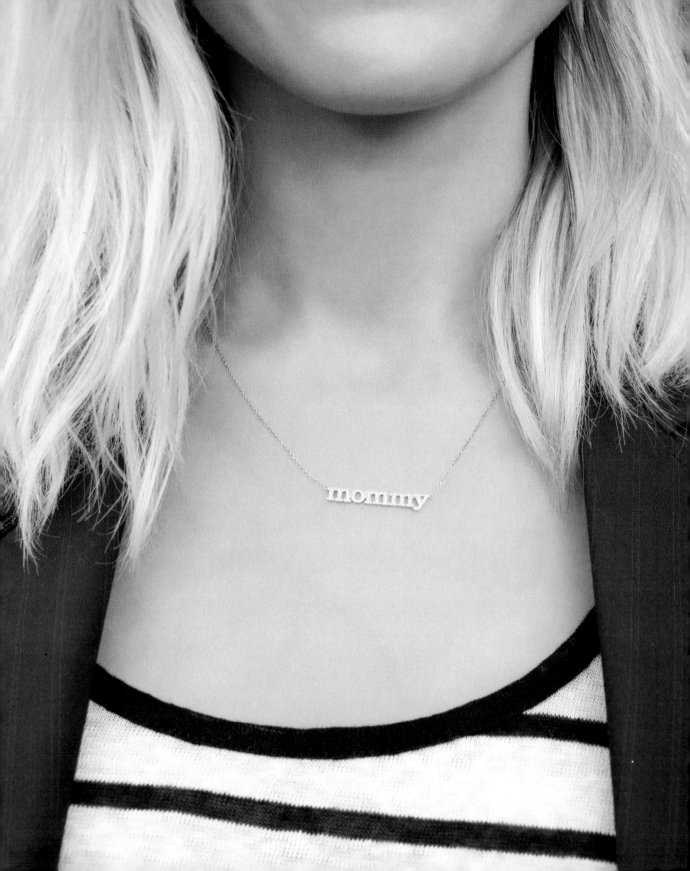

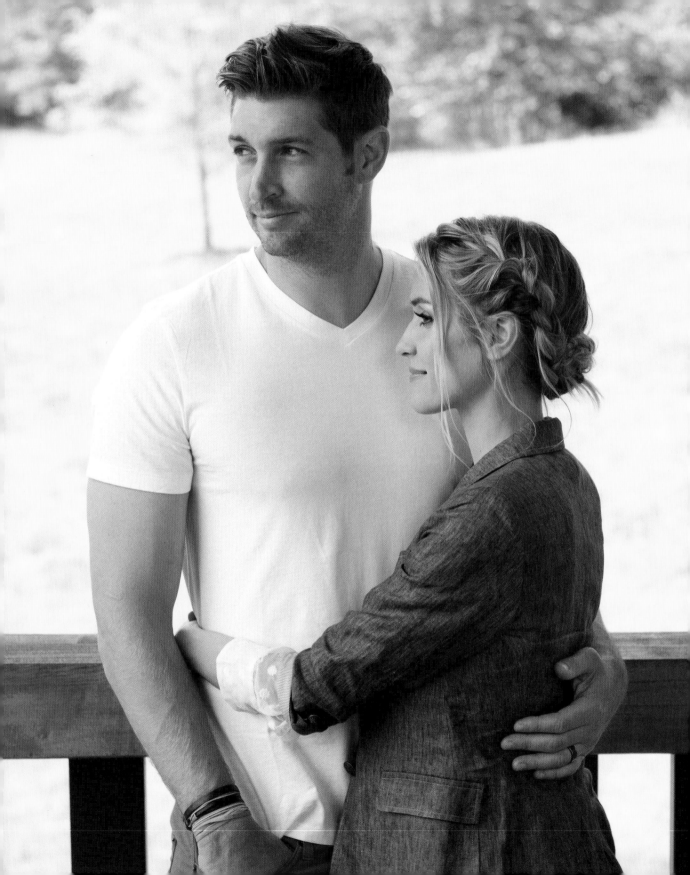

All Wifed Up

IF YOU WATCHED *LAGUNA BEACH*, THEN YOU SAW THAT AS A teenager, I came off as tough and like I had it all together, especially when dealing with the opposite sex. People asked me about this more than almost anything else regarding the show. "How do you have so much confidence when it comes to dealing with guys?" Well, I hate to break it to you, but that perceived confidence of mine wasn't the reality.

In fact, I was sort of a mess when it came to guys. Between being on a reality show and being a bit of a party girl, I had more than my share of romances that were either manipulated for TV or just plain bad for me. Luckily, my great love, Jay, came along right when I was ready to get serious. Now, I'm happily married to Jay and settled down with three kids—I even live in the suburbs! But it was a long road to get here, and I had tough lessons to learn along the way.

HIGH SCHOOL ROMANCE GONE WILD

I started at Laguna Beach High School my sophomore year, shortly after I moved to California from Illinois. I had a great boyfriend, Stephen, with whom I had a typical teenage romance. He was my entire world, and we loved hard and fought hard. Then in my junior year, after Stephen and I had been dating a little over a year (besides one short break), we were cast in MTV's show *Laguna Beach*. My relationship with Stephen went from our own high school romance to the fodder of a hugely successful television show.

Normal high school relationships are dramatic enough, but ours now had the added pressure of being seen by MTV viewers across the country as well as being manipulated by the show's producers, a set of adults who were suddenly very involved in the intricacies of our lives. Surprisingly, the producers had a bigger effect, as they controlled and mapped our lives more than we were aware. One of the most hurtful things they did was pressure Stephen to spend time with another girl from the show, Lauren, while he and I were dating. It certainly provided some juicy conflicts, but it also affected me deeply. I felt threatened. On one side, it seemed like the producers were trying to break us up, which was intimidating. On the other side, I worried that my relationship with Stephen was becoming less stable, even though I knew if we hadn't been on television, he wouldn't have been spending time with another girl. Because of all this, I did the only thing I knew how to do: put up a wall.

That made it look like I didn't care about anyone but myself. But Stephen was the most important thing in my life, and there was nothing I cared about more. I hated fighting with him on camera because it felt like I was airing all our dirty laundry. Even then, I knew that couldn't be good for a relationship. One time in particular, they showed me adamantly telling him, "I don't want to talk about it"—meaning, I didn't want to talk about whatever it was *on camera,* but it sounded as though I didn't want to deal with the issue at all. To some, I seemed confident and beyond my high school years; to others, I seemed like a mean girl. Either way, I

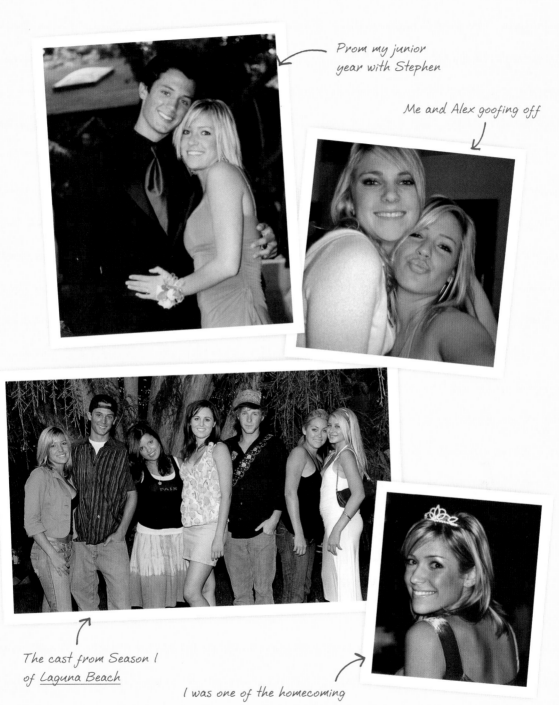

Prom my junior year with Stephen

Me and Alex goofing off

The cast from Season 1 of Laguna Beach

I was one of the homecoming princesses my senior year.

was shocked and sad that I was being portrayed as anything but myself: a sarcastic, goofy girl who just wanted to have fun.

The fact that I didn't take life too seriously and was a bit of a party animal didn't often put me in a good light. On a trip to Cabo San Lucas, when Stephen and I were actually broken up, I jumped up on the bar to dance with my girlfriends. Then I kissed a guy I was seeing at the time, completely unaware of how my actions were affecting Stephen (only teenagers are able to be so self-involved!). Not one of my better moments! Then Stephen started shouting "slut" at me from across the bar. It was a scene. There are certainly some clips I wish I could erase from everyone's memory.

But there are definitely times when the editing of the show exaggerated or misconstrued the reality. During that same trip to Cabo, I had to go to dinner with the cast—whom I wouldn't normally go to dinner with—and Stephen was mouthing "I love you" and being incredibly sweet to me even though we were broken up. But during editing, the producers made it seem like he was saying a lot of that to the other girl he was "seeing" and that I was rolling my eyes at him, which wasn't the case. Pretty deceptive! Producers also had Stephen go up to this same girl's house to hang out, which they made me believe was all on his own, so the joke was on me. Later I would find out they told him to go.

That said, I also didn't know how to deal with and handle my emotions. I was only 17! I had some anger stored up from my parents' divorce and my new stepfamilies, which the producers saw. They put me in situations where they knew

Advice I Wish I Had Given Myself

When in doubt, don't kiss someone for any of the following reasons:

▶ To make someone else jealous

▶ When you've had a little too much to drink

▶ Just because you are a big flirt and want attention!

I would react. I was a fighter back then: When I felt threatened, I acted. So when I felt the producers were trying to break up my relationship, I ended up becoming exactly what they wanted from the get-go. The only emotion I knew how to express was anger, which I didn't realize back then was just a cover for sadness and fear. When I acted out, they won.

One friend of mine, Alex, was always there for me. She filmed with me occasionally, which I loved because I was comfortable with her and she knew everything that was really going on with Stephen and me. We had a great friendship, always joking around and being silly together. Little moments of our goofiness—like the time we were doing the Miss America wave walking down her steps—came through on the show, which made us laugh when we saw it. She was someone I could turn to when I was upset.

Try not to get caught up in rumors or with the people who spread them. Deal with people face to face so you know what's real and what's not.

And luckily, what Stephen and I had together was real, and that's what made me get through the producers' attempt at manipulating us. We talked about everything the entire time. When we saw each episode, it was clear to us what was real and what was fake. We knew when a scene was edited to be seen differently than how it played out in real life, either by dubbing in words and implying you were talking about someone else to change the meaning of conversations, or by mixing scenes we'd filmed 5 months earlier with scenes we filmed the week before. But that still didn't make it easy. I think always having my guard up for those couple of years of filming made me reluctant to trust men.

GOTTA KISS A LOTTA FROGS

After high school, I dated some not-so-great guys. Looking back, I can boil it down to one thing: my lack of self-confidence. It took me awhile to grow up, love myself, and know my worth.

I know now that when you aren't happy with yourself, you put up with stuff you wouldn't normally accept. In my early twenties, I certainly let things slide and dated a few men who didn't give me the true respect that I deserved. I've always adored being in a relationship—I love having that connection and sharing your life with someone. But searching for a connection when your standards aren't what you *know* they should be can get you in trouble. I found myself with some people who lied right to my face and took advantage of me. I'm astonished sometimes when I think about the choices I made.

A couple of years before I met Jay, I dated one guy who, as it turned out, was seeing me in L.A. plus another girl in New York City the entire time. He was a powerful businessman, and I *knew* he wasn't a good guy. I had known him for years and saw what a jerk he was to women. But when we ended up having some business meetings and he turned on the charm, like an idiot I fell for it. He wined and dined me and said all the right words. He was *too* good. A girlfriend told me a story about him cheating on his ex-girlfriend, which she knew was true because she was friends with the ex. That still didn't stop me. My gut told me a thousand times to run the other way, but my insecurity kept me around for all of his BS. I'm just glad I had enough self-respect to end it with him after I found out about Ms. NYC. He showed up at my house begging to get me back, and I'm proud that I finally told him to hit the road.

Another guy actually *called* the paparazzi on us. I didn't figure this out until after we broke up. I honestly still look back and think, what an idiot I was! It was so obvious! Paparazzi would show up at the most random places when it was just the two of us. And *only* when it was just the two of us. This is one of the pitfalls of dating in L.A.—you can never trust that the person you are with wants you for you or for your ability to get them publicity. He even told me he called the paparazzi for another friend who briefly dated a celebrity, but I *still* didn't make the connection. Ugh!

A different fellow I dated made up all these stories about how crazy his ex was, and that he was so happy she was gone . . . blah, blah, blah. Then, while we were dating, I saw a picture on a blog of the two of them one weekend when he was in New York. Another guy sent flowers to me *and* another girl on Valentine's Day—we found out months later, when we ended up becoming friends completely independent of this guy. After we figured it out, we laughed and were glad he wasn't in either of our lives anymore. I also dated a man who always mooched off me. I paid for *everything*. I'm cool with paying for a lot of stuff, even half, but everything? I felt like his mom, and that was *not* sexy.

I knew those guys weren't good ones. My gut always told me something wasn't right, but I ignored it because, honestly, doing the right thing wasn't my priority then. I was in a party phase. I wasn't concerned with my long-term happiness. Looking back, I realize I was lonely and was searching for anything to hold on to.

I don't hate these guys or blame them. I truly believe you get what you put out there. Meaning, at the time, I wasn't really looking for Mr. Right. I was having fun and didn't want a serious boyfriend. Mix that with not loving myself, and those jerks were the men knocking at my door.

> If you are dating all the wrong guys, take a step back and look at yourself. Being comfortable with yourself and being able to express who you really are (like how you are with your family and friends) means that when the right person comes along, you'll be appreciated for you.

Looking back, I made plenty of excuses for these guys. I do wish I could have realized that if I thought he was lying, he probably was. That if he truly wanted to see me, he would make time—even at my busiest, I could *always* make time for someone I was interested in. There's a reason your gut is warning you and red flags are everywhere: Sometimes our bodies are more in tune with what's going on than our brains, especially when we have infatuation goggles on.

GROWING UP

I got to a point where I knew I wasn't truly happy and couldn't keep dating these men. During this time, I kept thinking back on one of my first boyfriends, before all the jerks. We were always laughing, he was incredibly sweet to me, but most important, I trusted him. He was crucial to my figuring out who I was. He always saw me in a better light than I saw myself and made me realize my potential. Simply, he made me feel good about myself. He told me I was the funniest girl he had ever met—and that meant a lot to me. He loved lighting candles, turning music on, and simply talking. He just wanted to know *me*. I was too young for that particular relationship, but I learned a lot from it in retrospect. When we were together, I was self-confident, secure, and authentically me. I realized those were the feelings I needed to get back.

I decided to focus on myself, to stop going out and hanging with a certain group of acquaintances, and to get my life together. I needed to start taking care of me. First, that meant figuring out who I was and what made me happy. I came face-to-face with my strengths and weaknesses and got real about my likes and dislikes. For example, I hate being vulnerable. Despite that, I want to be with someone who will take care of me. I can get angry quickly, which is something I still work on, and I have a tendency to assume things and see only my side. It took awhile to accept these things about myself. It felt like I decided to grow up.

Then I made an actual list of the qualities I wanted in a man. I listed "loyal" and "someone who I could ride in the passenger seat with." And I don't just literally mean to ride in the passenger seat with . . . in a broader sense, I wanted to feel

When in a relationship, it's also important to listen to your friends! If they warn you about the guy you're with, it's because they see something you don't. Friends know if someone is bringing us down . . . mine did! I wish I had listened much earlier.

protected and have the man take charge. I like things my way, but I wanted someone opinionated who wouldn't budge for everything I wanted. I didn't want him to care too much about his looks. Leave that part to me! Among other things, I also wrote that he had to be a good driver, have a nice chest and shoulders (had to include something physical!), like to have fun, and be secure and comfortable in his own skin.

It felt good to finally listen to my gut and get real about what I wanted in a man and what I wanted from myself.

OKAY, WORLD, I'M READY FOR MY HUBBY

After all this soul-searching, along came my future husband, Jay. The night before I met Jay, I actually tweeted, "I'm ready to meet my future boyfriend." Well, be careful what you wish for, because Jay checked off my entire list!

But the relationship didn't start out perfectly. You know how they say timing is everything? Well, I couldn't agree more. The first time I had heard of Jay was a year prior, when I had yet to do that growing up. When I was in the middle of filming *The Hills*, I got a phone call from my publicist saying that Jay Cutler wanted to fly me to Chicago and take me on a date.

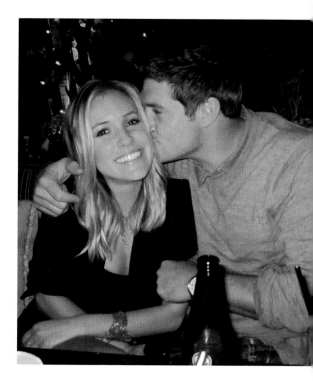

I always thought it was a funny thing to have your publicist call and tell you so-and-so wants to take you out. This person really knows nothing about you (he knows only your image, which isn't necessarily *you*), but he wants to give it a shot anyway. I always thought of this as a pretty ballsy move, like

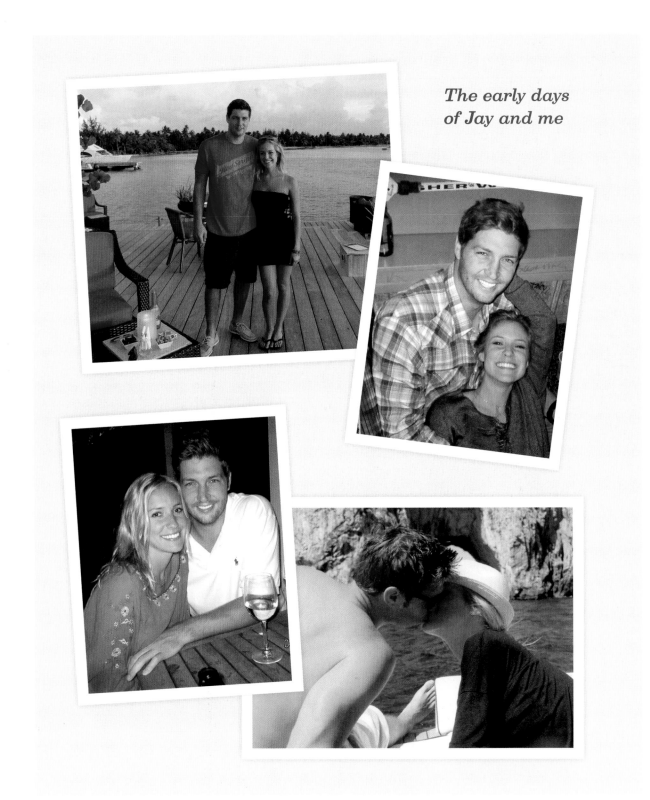

*The early days
of Jay and me*

you think very highly of yourself, and it turned me off a little. Plus, to be completely honest, years prior I had had a *different* Chicago athlete go through my publicist to ask me out, so I was a little weirded out by all these Chicago sports guys wanting to date me. I gotta give Jay some credit, though—later I found out it was another teammate responsible for the call, not Jay. Jay mentioned me to this other guy, who was trying to help Jay out. So at least Jay wasn't *that* egotistical!

I wasn't following football at that time, so I had never even heard Jay's name. My publicist told me he played football for the Chicago Bears, which still didn't help. So I googled Jay while we were on the phone. I thought he was cute, but I didn't take the request seriously and said no. I was living in L.A. at the time and busy with *The Hills*. Plus, I was still in party mode and not wanting a real boyfriend.

Cut to a year later, a year in which I grew up a lot and felt serious about meeting a good man (hence my tweet about it). I wanted out of the L.A. lifestyle— the clubbing and the superficial people. I had gone to visit my mom, who lives in a suburb of Chicago. We were going to a preseason football game with my Bears-obsessed cousin, Danny. I had completely forgotten about Jay asking me out until my mom brought it up on the way to the game, saying, "Kristin, didn't Jay Cutler ask you out?" "Um . . . did he? Yeah, I guess he did." At this moment in the conversation, I thought Danny was going to faint. He hadn't known about Jay's interest, and he thought I was insane for not going on a date. Thinking I would be cousin of the year, I called up my publicist and got us family passes to meet Jay after the game. Little did I know that I would end up marrying this man. When Jay walked into the room, I knew that instant. I got nervous and became shy, which only happens when I truly like someone.

> When Jay walked into the room, I knew that instant.

Mostly Jay talked to my mom and won her over. After a few minutes, he was polite enough to drive us to our car. We hung out 2 nights later, and that began a swift and intense romance. I flew back to Chicago at least every 2 weeks. When we were apart, we texted constantly, and he wrote me the sweetest love e-mails. He was the strong, manly man I wanted but had a sweet, romantic side as well.

He made me a priority, and we balanced each other out nicely, me being very outgoing and Jay more reserved. Jay told me he loved me weeks into our relationship and told me he wanted to marry me after only 2 months. It all happened quickly, but it made sense: He was exactly what I was looking for. I wanted a man, a real man. A guy who could fix something if it broke and whom I felt safe with, in every sense of the word. Eight months after our meeting came the ring.

Then, just 3 months later, I gave the ring back and called off the wedding.

Now let's back up for a minute. I always go after what I want in life, with men or otherwise, and I never settle. If something doesn't feel right, I act on it. It's just who I've always been. And at that moment, something wasn't right. A few things needed to change, and I knew the only way Jay would see how serious I was, was if I ended the relationship. On the outside, I tried to put on a tough, calm exterior even though I was dying on the inside. But that newly earned self-confidence and self-love made it possible to be that bold and to get myself through it. When you truly love yourself, you aren't afraid to walk away from a situation that isn't ideal, even if it means your heart will break. You take care of *you*. At least, that is what I told myself.

So I walked away from Jay, and it is the best thing that could have happened to our relationship. We talked the entire time we were broken up—working on a lot of things together—but I stuck to my guns.

One of the things we needed to resolve was my need to work. I've been working since I was 14. I'm naturally ambitious and driven—I got my first two jobs because

I wanted to, not because I had to. My dad is super-ambitious and self-made, which I respect. Everyone is different, but for me, working gives me confidence and independence, and those are things I need and treasure. I need creative outlets and something to call my own outside of family life. Jay comes from a pretty traditional background and envisioned himself being the sole breadwinner and his wife staying at home. But if I stayed home, I wouldn't be happy and would probably end up resenting Jay for it. We had butted heads about this since our relationship began, and I knew we had to hammer it out once and for all. We started seeing a therapist, whom I credit for saving our relationship. She opened up our eyes to the other person's perspective and gave us great tools for communication. Sometimes it takes an outsider to mediate and get things back on track. We still periodically see her to this day.

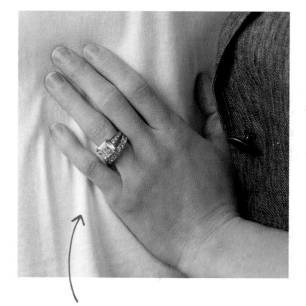

Jay picked out my engagement ring and wedding band by himself, no help from me!

After a long and difficult 2 months, we decided it was time to be together again, this time for good. I was still living in Los Angeles, but when I went to Chicago, I would stay for weeks at a time until I made the official move. We didn't fight like we did before. We had more compassion toward one another. I don't want you to think that all of a sudden everything was perfect, because it wasn't, and isn't. Jay and I still have problems, like all couples. Relationships are hard work, especially with kids. But those couple of months of being broken up showed us how much we meant to each other and how much we were both willing to do whatever it takes to make our relationship work.

THEN THERE WERE THREE

A couple of months after Jay and I got back together, we decided to try to get pregnant, and it worked. We were both thrilled, but telling Jay's parents was definitely nerve racking. They're a very traditional family, and I knew our having a baby on the way and not being married wouldn't sit well with them. While staying at their house on Christmas, we decided to break the news by wrapping up a printout of the ultrasound and putting it under the tree. Sure enough, the first thing Jay's mom said was, "Well, we're obviously going down to city hall to get married." Luckily, Jay did the talking and told his parents that just wasn't going to happen. They weren't pleased with our decision but still managed to be excited for us.

Honestly, at that point, even though I had a ring on my finger, part of me thought I still would never walk down the aisle. My parents divorced when I was 9, and between the stepfamilies and moving around, it was pretty difficult. I never wanted to put my kids through that. Also, I was perfectly happy being engaged the rest of my life. I knew Jay wasn't going anywhere. I already had that commitment from him and didn't need a piece of paper to give me security. The problem was, I knew Jay actually *did* want to get married. Part of me felt bad for him, but I also didn't want to do anything I wasn't ready for.

But then we had Cam, and everything changed. I started asking myself why I was against marriage. Having a kid made me realize that I wanted the security of a legal union for him. I wouldn't want him (or any of our kids, now) to ever interpret our voluntarily not getting married as a sign that Jay and I might not be completely committed to our family. I figured out that my reticence boiled down to one thing: my ego. Not marrying Jay gave me a false sense of control, as though I was in charge. But that wasn't what I actually wanted—I wanted the relationship to be fair and equal. Also, I felt as though not marrying Jay made me not give the relationship 100 percent; that not being married kept me from trying as hard as I could. I knew I wouldn't be all in unless we got married. Plus, we were in love and wanted to be together forever, so why not!

WEDDING BELLS

Once I came around to the idea of marriage, we wasted no time planning the wedding. When we first got engaged, before the breakup and Cam, the wedding we talked about was not us. It was huge, with nothing special or unique; it felt like we were settling, since everything about that ceremony was based on convenience and what everyone expected. Here's what's funny: The wedding we ultimately planned was the opposite of that. This time everything felt right. Our wedding really represented who we were: casual, intimate, and laid-back.

I found wedding planning to be fairly stress free. Overall, I tried to simply enjoy the process and prioritize what was most important. We wanted everyone to have a good time and remember the day, and we didn't want to have the same wedding as every other wedding you attend. We kept the event as small as possible (around 130 guests), set it in a place we loved, and kept the focus on the few things that mattered the most.

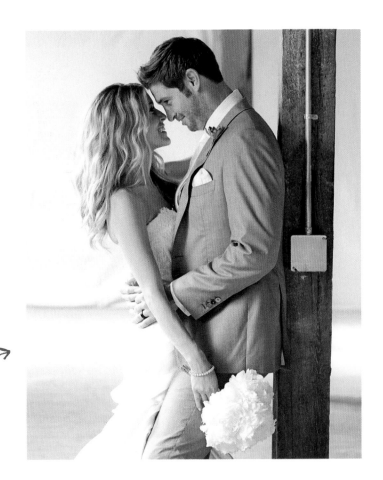

We were both on such a high after the ceremony! I felt like I was floating.

We wanted our wedding to be a fun party more than anything, so the most important item on our list was the music. Jay wanted to take the reins on this and spent hours on Web sites finding the perfect band. We wanted everyone dancing,

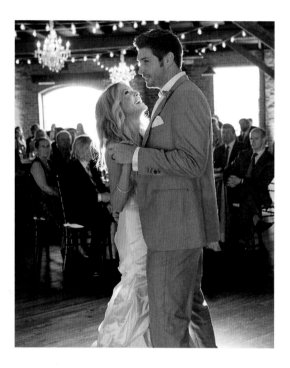

so we hired an awesome five-person Motown band. Next was the decor, which wasn't too difficult since I didn't want it to be too much. I wanted a clean, laid-back, rustic feel, so we put candles in mason jars and burlap on the tables and had minimal flowers. Nothing too perfect! My wedding planner nailed it—she couldn't have done a better job. And last, the food and booze were high on our list. We wanted everyone to have a memorable, authentic meal. We had upscale Southern comfort food—fried green tomatoes and pork sliders. And instead of doing a traditional Champagne toast, we gave everyone hard cider. That actually ended up being my drink of choice for the night, since it was light and refreshing and it was a hot summer night. Both Jay and I love Nashville (which is where Jay went to college and where we live half of the year), and we wanted our out-of-town guests to get the full Nashville experience and walk away loving it. Focusing on keeping it casual, intimate, and laid-back made everything easier. Nothing else seemed that important if we nailed those.

Everything went smoothly until that morning. I *thought* I was getting away with nothing going wrong, even though everyone always has that "one thing." Turns out I also had that one thing.

Our dog, Brando, was the sweetest 12-pound reddish-brown Maltipoo. He used to have separation anxiety, so whenever he got the chance, he would curl up in a ball on my neck and sleep for hours. This little guy was my dude. Or so I thought.

When planning a wedding, prioritize your list of to-dos and pick the top three things to make your priority. Wedding planning should be as stress-free as possible. Half the fun is the journey. So if the other things that don't matter as much aren't perfect, just let it roll off your back.

The morning of the wedding, I was at home with some family, playing on the floor with the kids and dogs. I put my head down by Brando, and next thing I know, I'm sitting up in pain, realizing that the hand I'm holding up to my face is covered in blood. Brando bit me right on the eye. Luckily, I closed my eye in time and he only got my eyelid. In shock, I went to a mirror. All I saw was a swollen eye and blood everywhere. I called Jay in hysterics, "You. Need. To. Get. Home. Right. Now." He could barely understand me through my sobbing. Later during his speech at the wedding, he would tell everyone, including me, that he thought I was calling off the wedding! Poor guy!

To make the situation weirder, I had scheduled a relaxing prewedding home yoga lesson. I tried to cancel, but the instructor insisted she knew Reiki and would be able to help. Looking for any solution, I agreed. After about 5 minutes of preliminary breathing and stretching, I told her I couldn't continue. My mind was *obviously* elsewhere and if she was gonna do Reiki, then we had to get on with it. So she moved her hand over my eye for about 15 minutes. And what do you know, my eye looked the same. In fact, it had gotten bigger. Luckily, my makeup artist is not only an angel but a freakin' magician. Karan walked in after my failed Reiki session and immediately said, "It's not that bad!" She didn't seemed fazed at all and instead got to work like any other day. She literally glued my cuts closed with eyelash glue and worked some serious magic. My right eye looked a little smaller than my left when all was said and done, but honestly, you couldn't tell. I'm a big believer in everything happening for a reason and that there's a lesson to be learned in everything . . . but to this day, I have absolutely no clue why that happened! Jay says maybe it was for him, because even though he was already madly in love, it made him appreciate me even more.

Besides that blip, the day was truly perfect. All of the speeches were amazing—my maid of honor and Jay's best man had us falling out of our seats. My dad and stepdad both gave incredibly heartwarming toasts, and Jay had me in tears as he poured his heart out in his speech. I still have his note cards, which I keep in a special place to go back and read occasionally. The band had the crowd dancing, everyone mentioned how great the food and decor were, and we had a hilarious photo booth with accessories (oversize sunglasses, hats) for people to goof off in. Those pictures made for great memories! Most important, we were able to talk to everyone that night and still enjoy each other.

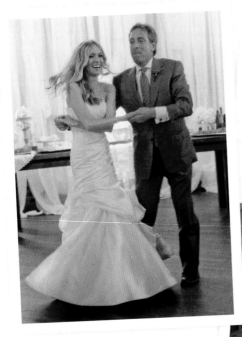

One of the best days of my life

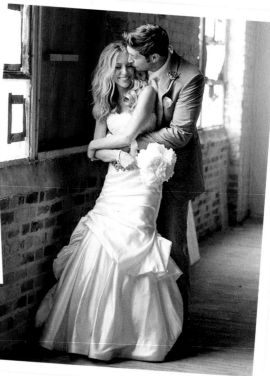

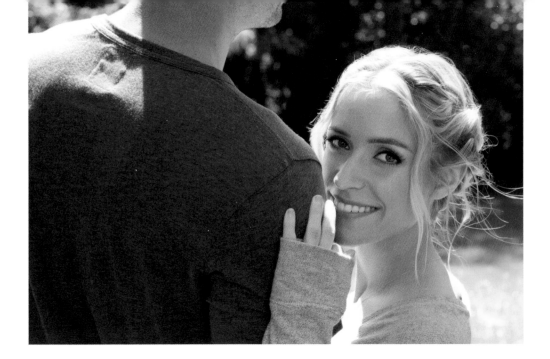

MARRIED LIFE

Nothing practical really changed after we got married. We already lived together and had a baby, so most typical newlywed things had been checked off by the time we said "I do." But mentally, it was different. Being married pushed me out of my comfort zone. Now it was real! I couldn't leave when we fought. I couldn't just say I was done. I had to emotionally grow up. I had to become aware of my needs and learn how to express them. If this relationship was going to work, then I had to become a better fighter (and maybe less of a fighter, for that matter).

Our minister gave me a book called *The Five Love Languages*. While reading it on our honeymoon, a lightbulb went off. Holy shit! I finally figured us out! The book describes five different "languages" that people use in love relationships—ways that we express love and feel love. "Affirmation" was certainly 100 percent me: needing to hear I am loved, which Jay isn't the best at (sorry, babe!). Instead, Jay shows his love by doing things *for* me, like putting gas in my car without my asking or making dinner for my girlfriends and me, known as "acts of service" in the book. But when Jay shows his love to me through *his* love language, it doesn't mean as much to me since that's not how *I* feel love. Same goes for me—if I tell Jay I love him, it doesn't register like it would if I *did* something for him. We were lying by the

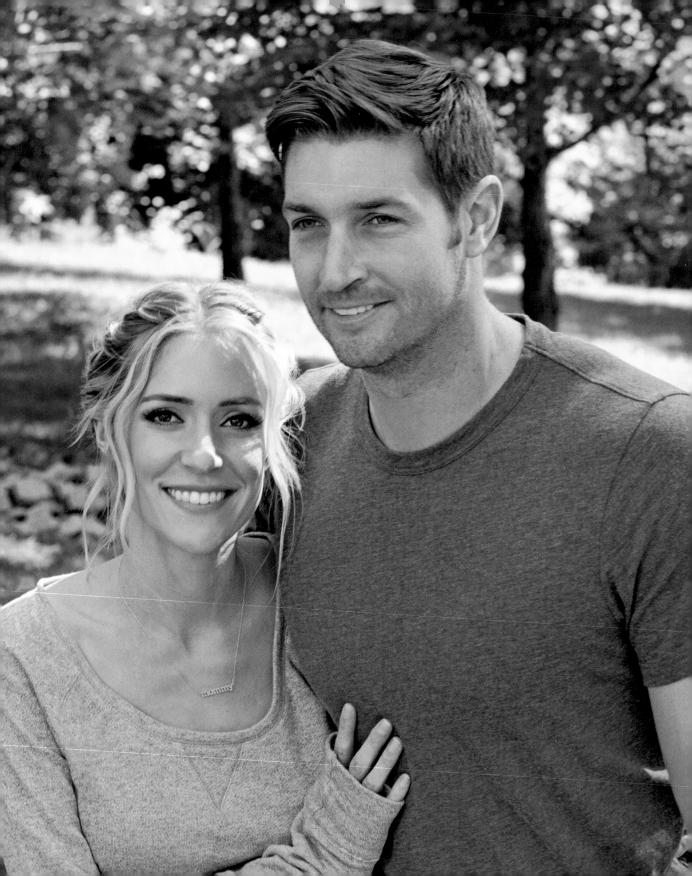

pool on the Amalfi coast when I was reading the book, and I still hadn't figured out Jay's language when he needed to run up to the room to grab something. Before he left he asked me to order him a drink. But the server never came around, so I didn't order it. When I saw how upset Jay was over my not getting him a drink, I almost fell out of my chair. Acts of service! These things now seem so obvious, but they had never crossed my mind until this book came along.

Whether you read that book or not, it's crucial to know what you need and what your partner needs in a relationship. If you are lost, how is someone else supposed to help? Communication is the foundation of our relationship, especially after our breakup. I'm glad to be in a relationship where I feel safe expressing my needs. I used to assume my boyfriends knew how I was feeling and what I needed from them. I even found myself in the beginning assuming that Jay knew what I was feeling. I had to learn how to identify and express my thoughts better. Further, it's hard to fix something if you don't know it's broken. I have one girlfriend who is miserable in her relationship but has never vocalized that to her husband. How in

Communication Makes Everything Better

Seeing a therapist has improved our relationship dramatically. We can put ourselves in the other person's shoes now, and we've learned how to talk about things without being hurtful. Good communication skills are everything.

▶ Say "I," not "you." Talk about how something made *you* feel, instead of assigning the other person the blame by saying "You did this" or "You did that."

▶ Never say "but." As in, "You're great at this, *but* you did that."

▶ Validate the other's feelings.

▶ Don't stonewall, have contempt for, or criticize the other person, or be defensive.

▶ Try to be curious about how the other person is feeling and have empathy.

▶ Always have a positive intention going into an intimate conversation.

the world are things going to get better if he thinks everything is fine? It's not fair to you, the other person, or the relationship.

There is no doubt that relationships are hard work. I would love to sit here and say that things with Jay and me are always perfect, that all we do is laugh and never fight. I know those couples (at least the ones that put on that front), and I'm not afraid to admit that we're definitely not one of them. Relationships take energy and commitment, and you can never get complacent. Relationships are ever changing because people change. My relationship with Jay is an entirely different one than our first year together. It's different today from when we first had Camden and Jaxon, and now with three kids. It's always evolving. And for us, it's getting better, in the sense that we are figuring each other out and learning how to make the other person happy. We have our fights, and I still shed some tears occasionally, but I'm proud to say we've gotten *better* at fighting. Our arguments don't escalate like they used to, and we rebound more quickly—we know that we are on the same team and working toward the same goal. When we broke up, it made us both realize we didn't want to be apart and we were willing to do whatever it takes to make it work. Marriage to me is about the act, over and over again, of making it work.

STAYING CONNECTED WHEN YOU'RE APART

Even not being together can be meaningful if you make an effort. I actually love traveling for work because it makes me miss Jay. I can't wait to see him. I get excited to come home and hug him after being gone for a couple of days. I still get little butterflies in my stomach. Here is what we do the days we are apart.

- Video call each other constantly. It helps a lot to see the person you miss so much! Thank God for technology.

- Send sexy pictures. I always cut my head out, though. You can never be too careful!

- I've been known to sext from time to time. Gotta do whatcha gotta do! Even if it means you are doing five other things at the same time and just going along with it for your man. ;)

Easy Ways to Get Hubby Time In

Both of our schedules are crazy, and during the football season it can be hard to carve out quality alone time. I need to feel connected and on the same page as Jay; otherwise, everything feels thrown off. Since I know this about myself, I try to make date night a priority. It doesn't happen as often as we would both like (ideally, we would have it once a week), but when it does come together, it's great.

DATE NIGHT OUT: I always feel great when we get dressed up and go out for dinner or even just a drink. It brings me back to the early days of our relationship.

DATE NIGHT AT HOME: If I can't find a sitter, I like to cook an elegant dinner after the kids go to bed (see "Date Dinners for You and Your Hubby" on page 110 for some ideas), open a bottle of wine, light some candles, and put our phones away.

TAKE A BATH TOGETHER: This doesn't even have to be sexual! It's more about connecting. I like adding a few drops of rose essential oil.

PUT ON SOME LINGERIE: Sometimes it's all you need. It makes me feel sexy and changes things up!

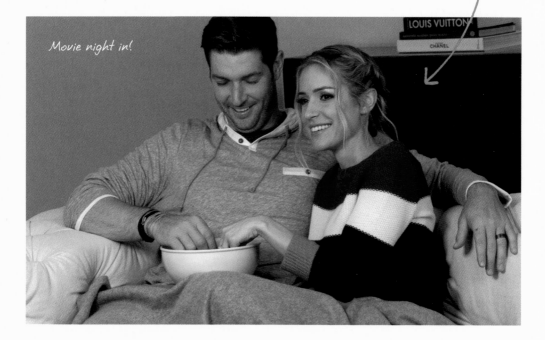

Movie night in!

THE IMPORTANCE OF FRIENDSHIPS

Friendships are similar to romantic relationships in the sense that they need nurturing; they need time and energy to sustain themselves and grow. It's easy to get caught up in work and kids and husbands and realize it's been awhile since we've spoken to our friends. But it's important to balance partner time and time with friends. I think it's healthy for Jay to hang with the guys and me with the girls. I want Jay to go have a good time without my giving him a hard time about it. We each need to blow off steam and enjoy those moments. There's nothing attractive about having a leash on your spouse. Plus, I've noticed it actually makes the person pull further away.

I would be lost without my girlfriends. Remember when we were younger and everyone kept telling us that as we got older we would have fewer and fewer friends? Boy, were they right. I can count my *good* friends on one hand, and I'm happy about that because they are all great girls. It's true what they say: quality over quantity!

My girls bring so much joy and laughter to my life. I cherish the time I have with them, especially since it isn't as often as I'd like anymore. Half of my good friends live in L.A., but when we make the effort to see each other (either they visit me, or I stay an extra day or two after a business trip), it's as though no time has passed. I can truly be my bubbly, goofy self with them. We enjoy the same things—fashion, traveling, reading, health—and could talk, joke around, and laugh for hours. We are also shoulders for one another to cry on, to vent to, and to bitch to. They get things that guys don't understand: small things like how we're stressing about the fine lines on our face or if the latest trend is worth spending money on, and bigger stuff like how we handle our emotions. I need that!

Plus, like Jay, my girls never judge me or make me feel bad about myself, but they aren't afraid to call me out when I'm not making the best decision or I'm being an idiot. Nothing I love more! *That* is a true friend right there. I also don't want a friend who is a yes-man (yes-woman?) and automatically agrees with everything I say or do. I want my friends to be their own persons and have minds of their own. I rely on my good friends to be honest and to voice their opinions when they disagree with me. I don't want the type of friend who tells you your jeans look great when we all know they look like shit. Be real with me. Don't tell me you love my boyfriend just to tell me what I want to hear. I want the truth. And I will give the truth right back to you, since that's what I value in other people.

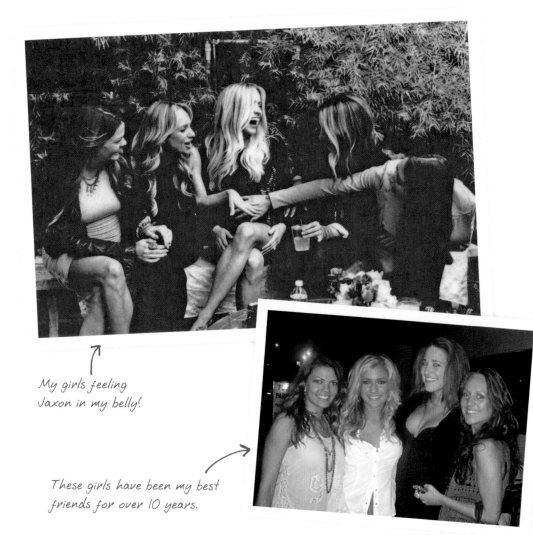

My girls feeling Jaxon in my belly!

These girls have been my best friends for over 10 years.

Balancing It All

Being in a successful relationship requires balancing your love and understanding for another person with your love and understanding for yourself. Once I was able to have the confidence to define what I wanted and needed and to believe that I deserved that, I was able to meet and marry someone as incredible as Jay.

Jay is my family, and family is the most important thing to me. We do have to consciously make time for the relationship, though, for just Jay and me. When I was living in Los Angeles, we used to have a "no more than 2 weeks" rule—and to date, we've never gone more than 2 weeks without seeing each other. Since we've had kids, it's closer to 3 days. (The only exception is training camp, but Jay has every fifth day off and comes home. Now that Cam and Jax are older, I'm going to take them to him for a few days every year.)

Balancing your relationship also means making the effort for each other and doing things that are right for the team. Getting married after having a kid felt like the best decision I could make for my family, and I'm so glad I did. I try to always make a nice dinner and do the laundry, since I know those go a long way with Jay. When he makes the effort to write me a note, even just a stickie note placed on my pillow saying he loves me, it literally makes my whole world. And every day we are together, we hug and kiss periodically throughout the day. Sometimes it's the little things that make a world of difference.

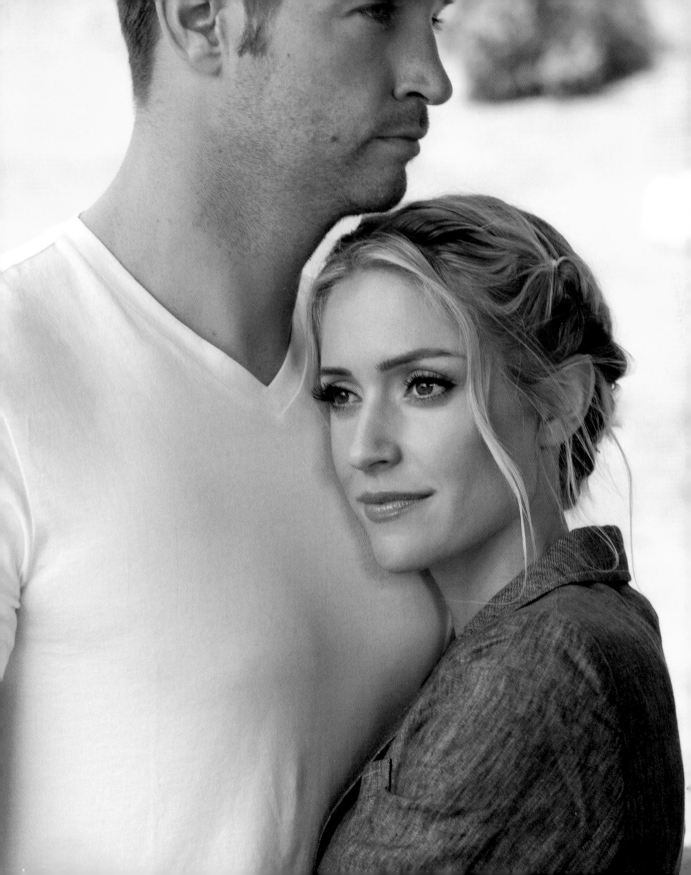

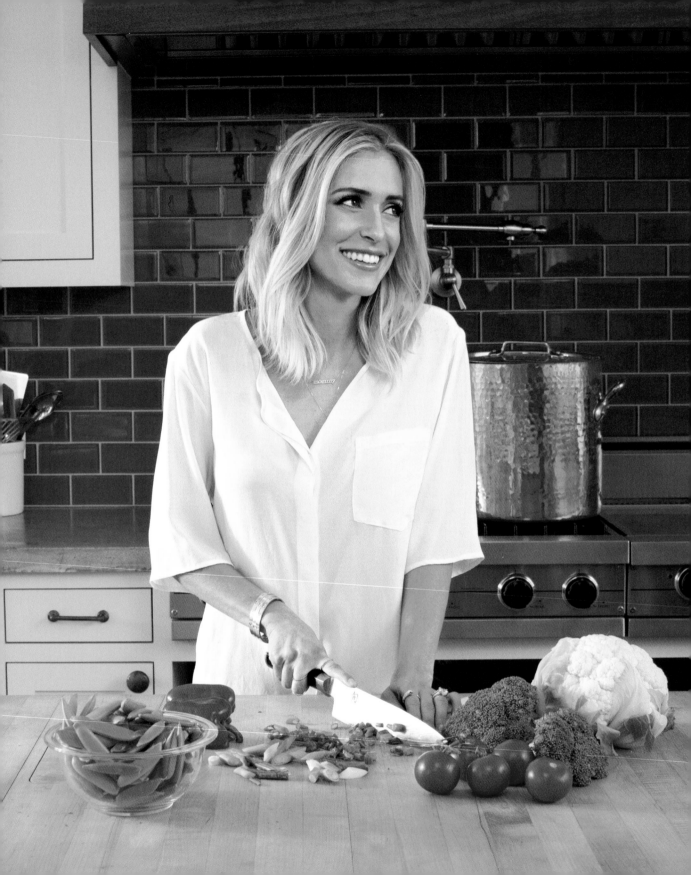

You Are What You Eat

MY DIET AND MY RELATIONSHIP WITH FOOD HAVE CHANGED
drastically over the years. In my late teens and early twenties, I was
a serious calorie counter and was always thinking about my weight.
While I obsessed over eating only low-calorie and low-fat food, I
never thought about the actual content of what I was putting in my
body. When I became pregnant at 24, everything changed. Now I
don't even glance at calories, and I've never felt healthier. It's taken
me a long time to get here, but my philosophy these days is simple
and permanent: Avoid artificial ingredients and strive to eat only
real food.

LOSING WEIGHT ALL THE WRONG WAYS

For years, I bought into the idea that zero-calorie and low-fat foods are good for you and will help you lose weight. Occasionally, I'd try another diet. You name it, I've done it: the Zone Diet, no-carb diet, grapefruit diet. There was even one period when I would eat a block of cheese and justify it by saying I was on the Atkins diet. Ha! But primarily, as early as high school, I thought that depriving myself of certain foods (sweets and carbs) and limiting calories would result in the body of my dreams. I had cartons of Splenda in my apartment to put on everything. If a box said "low fat"—cookies, cereals, TV dinners—I was buying it. Since I thought that healthy eating was based strictly on number of calories, my diet included all kinds of processed, prepackaged foods, often the ones marketed to girls like me. I never thought twice about where my food was coming from or if it was made in a lab.

Beyond the food itself, my eating habits were equally damaging. I would be super-strict for 5 days, then binge eat for 2. During the week, I tried to stay around 1,800 calories a day and would be hungry and unsatisfied most of the time. Then the weekend came, and it was a free-for-all. I drank numerous vodka cranberries and ate everything I didn't allow myself the previous 5 days. Grilled cheese, pizza, fries dipped in ranch dressing, red velvet cupcakes, and ice cream were on the menu, and all at the same time. I remember times when one girlfriend and I would order enough delivery food to feed eight people, and we would polish it all off. Then, come Monday, I was back to eating salads and low-fat diet food. Talk about horrible for your body! It's safe to say I didn't have a great relationship with food.

During this time, I never lost weight. My skin was never clear, the whites of my eyes didn't glow, and I always had a "pooch" that I could never shed. I didn't have a ton of energy either. I did notice a difference when I would go through short periods of drinking an occasional green juice (different vegetables juiced with an apple and lemon) and eating organic food: I felt better and even looked a little healthier. But then I always ended up going back to eating crap.

MY TURNING POINT

It wasn't until I became pregnant with my first son, Camden, that I realized something had to change. I wanted the best for my baby and knew that everything I was eating was going right to him. Low-fat cookies and processed junk were not what I'd feed a baby, so I didn't want to feed them to him in utero either. I was responsible for his well-being, and I certainly didn't want to jeopardize his health. Because of the small boost I felt when I ate more whole foods, I thought there might be something to the organic, natural lifestyle. Before being pregnant, trying a new diet was always a bit scary, as I never knew if it would result in what I wanted—but this time, I was not concerned about my weight at all, which was freeing. So I set off on what would become an odyssey into research, and I was lucky enough to consult with my incredible integrative doctor, Sam Moltz, MD.

After wading knee-deep in information, I found the consensus is that we have a ton of artificial chemicals in our food supply that are extremely harmful to our health. I avoid genetically modified organisms (GMOs) because they've been banned (or at least labeled) in more than 60 countries, and we haven't studied the long-term effects they have on the body. GMOs are linked to digestive problems, among other things. Antibiotics and growth hormones are other additives being excessively pumped into the animals we are eating, which means we're then consuming those excess antibiotics and hormones. And some processed foods actually contain toxic chemicals, often used to prevent spoilage and enhance flavor. I truly believe that everything I need to flourish nutritionally is found in nature and that some stuff just shouldn't be messed with, especially the food I'm putting in my body. After learning about all of these "extras" in our food, it scared the you-know-what out of me.

> I truly believe that everything I need to flourish nutritionally is found in nature and that some stuff just shouldn't be messed with, especially the food I'm putting in my body.

There was no way I wanted my baby to be consuming these scary foods, and certainly not because of my habits. I decided not to look at calories anymore; from that point, I focused on the ingredient label—and often the new food I ate (like fruits and veggies) didn't have an ingredient label at all! I ate only real, whole foods, nothing highly processed, and nothing potentially harmful to my health. This meant I could now eat pasta, cheese, and ice cream, as long as the ingredients were real. I didn't put a limit on myself; if I wanted something, I had it. I could eat whatever I wanted and however much I wanted, as long as what I put in my mouth was real food. I didn't care how much weight I gained. I wanted to enjoy pregnancy, to give my baby the best start possible, and not worry about the number on the scale.

I gained only 25 pounds during my pregnancy. I was shocked and knew there had to be something to this new eating approach. I didn't feel deprived, I was always satisfied, and I finally had a healthy relationship with food. I ate more than I ever did and managed not to blow up. I decided to maintain this healthy lifestyle, and 5 years later, I've never had to diet. My skin looks the best it ever has, and my energy has soared. Even getting sick is now a thing of the past—and not just for me, but for my entire family.

A NEW FOOD PHILOSOPHY

People think that because I'm "healthy," I'm missing out on life and never eat sweets or carbs. But you are talking about a girl with the biggest sweet tooth. I've been like that since I was little; I could eat ice cream for breakfast. (As a matter of fact, I used to save my leftover Dairy Queen mint chip Blizzards and do just that.) My life is quite the opposite of what people might think. I eat everything I want . . . burgers, pasta, cake, you name it. I'm no longer missing out, and I'm actually enjoying food. It's no longer a mental battle about "if I eat this, then I'll gain that much weight." I'm the freest I've ever been regarding what I put in my body.

That said, I do stay away from cow's milk. A food sensitivity test concluded that I am highly sensitive to casein, the main protein in cow's milk. I was okay with

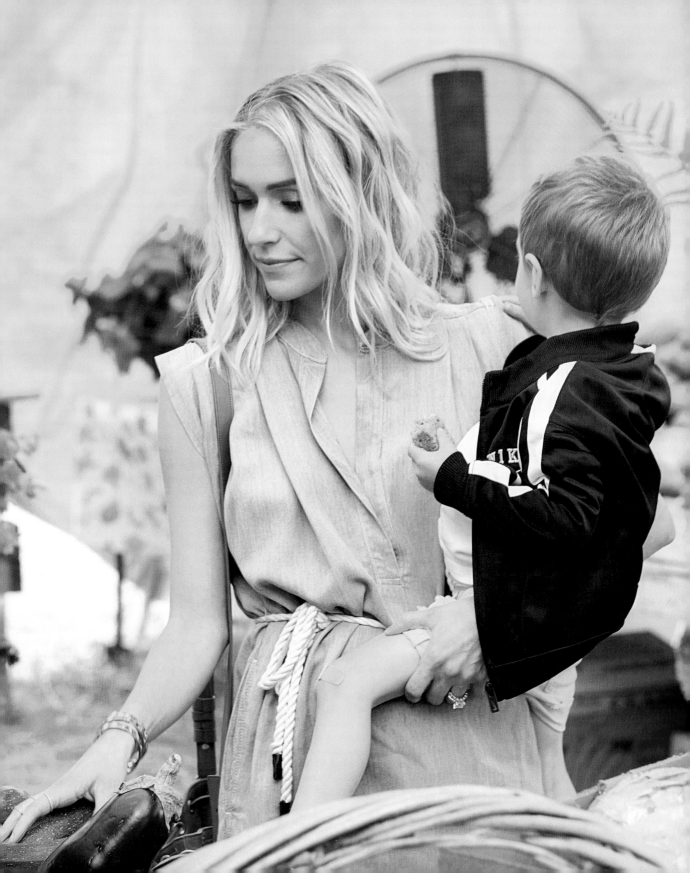

that diagnosis because most commercial cow's milk today is full of growth hormones and antibiotics. No, thanks. Instead, I drink almond or coconut milk. They are both so tasty that I never miss dairy milk. Plus, I can still eat all the buffalo's, sheep's, and goat's milk cheeses I want, which in general are much easier on the digestive system since they are lower in casein (and contain different types of casein) than cow's milk.

So what exactly does all this mean? It's simple: When I am eating at home, our food is as clean as can be. This means mostly whole foods: organic as often as possible, wild-caught fish, and grass-fed beef. I'm aware of where my meat is coming from. If it's been pumped full of antibiotics and growth hormones, I stay away. As much as possible, we eat foods that are not (or are only minimally) processed, and we select food that is nutrient dense and real. When it comes to the processed food I cannot avoid (like coconut milk, pasta, and nut butters), it means that I've become a psycho about reading every single ingredient label and researching the ingredients I don't recognize. I've ultimately realized that eating well should be a lifestyle, a consistent, realistic approach to food. Food is no longer about a diet or quick fix.

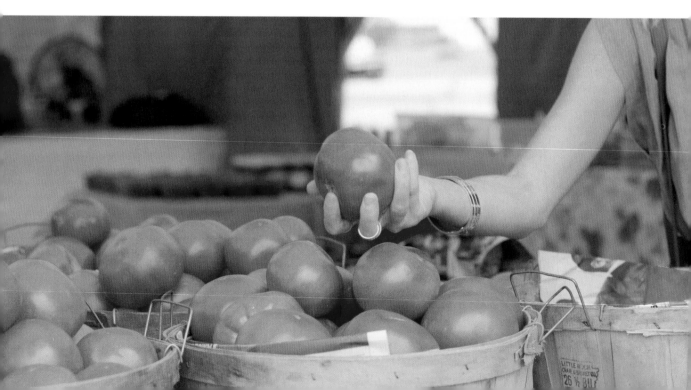

WHAT TO EAT AND WHAT TO WATCH OUT FOR

Unfortunately, particular qualities of our food supply have gone rapidly downhill in the last 20 years. We now have chemicals in our food that other countries have banned. We pump our cows full of antibiotics and hormones to produce more meat and milk. Then we feed our livestock a diet of GMOs, so they aren't getting the best nutrition either. All of that garbage is then being ingested by us. It's unfortunate that clean eating is seen as something of a luxury rather than what's normal. Here is a breakdown of what I watch for and why.

Avoiding GMOs

Did you know that more than 70 percent of processed food contains genetically modified organisms? These are organisms whose genetic material has been altered using genetic engineering techniques. Some people will argue that GMOs are necessary for good plant breeding, that they are just an extension of natural hybridizing or selective breeding. Certain crops, such as wheat, can naturally hybridize in nature. But for this to happen, the crops have to be the same species or closely related forms. GMOs today are made in a lab by combining completely different species and DNA. They don't organically occur in nature. Unless created by man, they would never exist.

These days, there are three major types of genetically modified (GM) foods. The first is known as *Bt*. Plants with this toxin have been given a built-in pesticide. When a bug eats the crop (often corn, cotton [for oil], and soy), its stomach explodes and it dies. That toxin—that makes bugs explode—is what we are eating. Scary. To me, that doesn't seem perfectly safe. The second type of GM food is Roundup Ready. This crop is made to withstand the herbicide Roundup, which is used in commercial farming to kill certain weeds and grasses. No matter how much Roundup you spray, the crop will not die. This is supposedly good for farmers, who want a high yield of the crop in question, but the problem is, everything else around it dies: worms, the good bacteria in the soil, and nutrient-rich weeds. (Nutrient-rich weeds are important because when they die naturally, their minerals are released back into the soil. Without nutrient-dense soil, our crops don't have as much nutritional value when we eat them.) Plus, Roundup still soaks into the plant, and there are concerns that residues remain even after you wash the fruits and vegetables harvested from those plants. Roundup contains a chemical called glyphosate that destroys human gut bacteria needed for a healthy immune system. Glyphosate has been labeled a probable carcinogen by the International Agency for Research on Cancer. Yikes. The third type of GM foods is a crop that's been injected with a promoter, which is used to introduce foreign DNA to achieve a desired trait, such as a certain color. Personally, I'm more interested in my food (and other things, for that matter) being natural rather than looking perfect.

At the very least, I wish we labeled foods with GMOs here in the States like other countries do. If biotech companies are so proud of their GM products, then what are they afraid of? Why are they spending *millions* of dollars lobbying to *not* have them labeled? I think we have a right to know what we are feeding ourselves and our children. If GM foods were labeled, then each person could make his or her own decision on whether to consume them.

COMMON GMOS

Here are some plants that commonly contain GMOs, unless they are labeled "organic" or "Non-GMO Project Verified."

- ▸ **APPLES**

- ▸ **CANOLA OIL** (used in many products like chips, premade chicken salad, and fake butter)

- ▸ **CORN** (Make sure to read labels, because corn is an ingredient in many things, including chips, baking powder, and vanilla.)

- ▸ **COTTON** (cottonseed oil)

- ▸ **HAWAIIAN PAPAYA**

- ▸ **POTATOES**

- ▸ **SOYBEANS** (Soy is in many products you wouldn't think of, such as protein bars and chocolate. Watch out for soy lecithin and soy isolates.)

- ▸ **SUGAR BEETS**

- ▸ **YELLOW SQUASH**

- ▸ **ZUCCHINI**

Chemicals in Surprising Places

There are thousands of chemicals allowed in our food, some worse than others, but there are a few that I absolutely avoid, no matter what. You will never see me eat anything containing **HIGH FRUCTOSE CORN SYRUP**. Some studies suggest it drives people to overeat and gain weight plus causes a multitude of health issues like heart disease.

If a food contains **SYNTHETIC DYES** (such as FD&C blue, green, and yellow artificial colors), I won't touch it. In years past, other colors made it into our food supply and were later taken off the shelves because of the harm they were proven to cause. Why are today's colors magically safe, and how do we know they won't be proven otherwise in 10 years?

ARTIFICIAL SWEETENERS (aspartame, saccharin, acesulfame K, and sucralose) are known to alter gut flora and may contribute to obesity instead of helping people lose weight. This is why diet drinks, in my eyes, are actually worse for you than a regular drink made with sugar.

BUTYLATED HYDROXYANISOLE (BHA) and **BUTYLATED HYDROXYTOLUENE (BHT)** are preservatives that prevent spoilage and keep food from changing color and flavor, and BHA is potentially cancer causing. Yikes . . . not normal. Food is supposed to spoil, not be able to live on a shelf for years. **SODIUM NITRATES** and **SODIUM NITRITES** are preservatives found in processed meats, bacon, lunchmeats, and hot dogs. You can find these food items without those preservatives, but you have to read the labels carefully.

MONOSODIUM GLUTAMATE (MSG) is a flavor enhancer and has been shown to alter brain chemistry. MSG gives some people a headache within minutes of eating it. **POTASSIUM BROMATE** is an additive used to increase volume in some white flour, breads, and rolls and may cause cancer in animals. **BROMINATED VEGETABLE OIL (BVO)** is banned in other countries and is used as an additive for gasoline. Yummy. Sports drinks, which used to be my go-to hangover cure and probably just made me feel worse, are one place where you can find BVO. **SODIUM BENZOATE** and **POTASSIUM BENZOATE** can be hard to avoid, but they can worsen allergies in people who are sensitive to them and create digestive issues.

And last but not least, **SODIUM SULFITE**. This is a preservative used in making wine and other processed foods. Do you ever get a massive headache while drinking wine? I'm not talking about a hangover, I'm talking a pounding headache after one glass. It probably means you are allergic to the sulfites. I know many people who have this issue. One person in a hundred is sensitive to sulfites in food and wine, so the reaction is fairly common. Other symptoms besides a headache are a rash and/or breathing problems that can be especially problematic if you have asthma. Pretty scary stuff, huh? And these few chemicals are just the tip of the iceberg.

All of this can feel incredibly overwhelming. At first, it seems like there's absolutely no way you can avoid all of these chemicals, and you may want to give up. Here's what you do: Start small. You eliminate one thing at a time until it becomes second nature. So, for example, start with added colors. They are fairly easy to spot and not impossible to give up. For a few weeks, whenever you go to the grocery store, read the ingredient label anytime you pick up a food item. If you see added colors (FD&C Red 40, Yellow 5, and Blue 1), don't buy it. That's it. Not too hard. Then, once you notice added colors and you automatically pass on those food products, add another chemical you want to avoid. Keep going until you are a pro at reading labels. I promise that eventually it will be easy. I still don't know what every chemical is, but I know which ones I definitely don't want to eat, and they stick out like a sore thumb. Also, the great thing is, eventually if you stay away from processed food altogether, you won't have to worry about these added ingredients.

> All of this can feel incredibly overwhelming. . . . Here's what you do: Start small. You eliminate one thing at a time until it becomes second nature.

Hidden Additives

I can't stress enough the importance of reading labels on every packaged food you buy. Added colors, dairy, soy, and more are in everything from cereal to pharmaceutical drugs. Read the ingredient label so you can avoid what you want to avoid. Some chemicals are worse than others, and even though I try to avoid the majority of them, occasionally a few get by. It's nearly impossible to never eat an added chemical, but I always look for the least amount of ingredients in a food as possible. Would you have thought that the following items can contain these additives?

VITAMINS: added colors, carrageenan (a controversial chemical), maltodextrin (usually GM unless organic or non-GMO verified), titanium dioxide (filler), nickel (a known carcinogen). Try to purchase vitamins with the fewest added ingredients, around three or four max.

COOKING SPRAYS: soy (typically GM unless organic or non-GMO verified)

VINEGARS: caramel color

PACKAGED NUTS/TRAIL MIX: MSG, modified cornstarch (typically GM)

GUM: aspartame. I buy two brands that don't include any scary ingredients: Glee Gum and Spry gum. Unfortunately, the flavor doesn't last as long, but at least you have peace of mind that you aren't chewing something bad for your health!

PICKLES: artificial dyes (FD&C Yellow 5), preservatives (sodium benzoate)

MEDICATIONS (PRESCRIBED AND OVER THE COUNTER): added colors, BHA, wax, talc. There may not be much you can do about this, but it's something to be aware of.

Eating Organic

I believe in eating organic as often as possible. Nonorganic fruits and vegetables are sprayed with numerous pesticides that don't always wash off; I don't want those pesticides in my system. When you buy organic meat, it means the livestock wasn't given GM feed and wasn't pumped full of antibiotics and growth hormones. Huge upside! Understandably, it can be hard to access or afford an all-organic diet. One way to make eating organic easier is by becoming familiar with the Environmental Working Group's Dirty Dozen and Clean Fifteen. The Dirty Dozen are 12 fruits and vegetables that have the highest amount of pesticides, so they are the ones to buy organic if possible. The Clean Fifteen are the ones with the lowest amounts of pesticides, making the conventional/nonorganic options okay to eat. It's important to frequently check the lists, since they vary annually. Another technique is to buy produce in season and directly from farmers' markets. Local produce is more nutrient rich (and delicious) since it didn't have to travel as far, plus in-season produce is often less expensive than out-of-season produce. Bonus: Local produce is better for the environment since less transport is necessary.

CLEAN FIFTEEN

You can feel fine about not buying organic versions of the following veggies and fruits:

1. Asparagus
2. Avocados
3. Cabbage
4. Cantaloupe
5. Cauliflower
6. Eggplant
7. Grapefruit
8. Kiwifruit
9. Pineapples
10. Mangoes
11. Onions
12. Papaya (could be a GMO, though!)
13. Sweet corn
14. Sweet peas (frozen)
15. Sweet potatoes

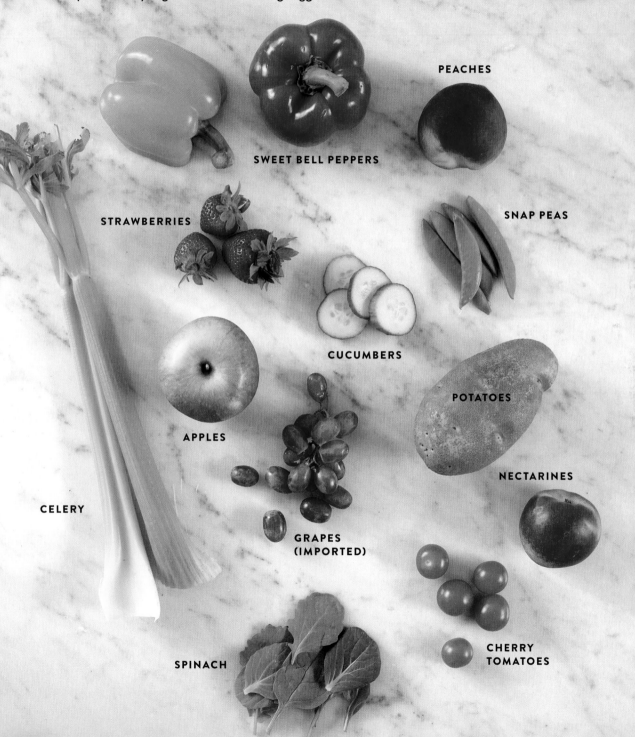

Dirty Dozen

When possible, buy organic for the following veggies and fruits:

SWEET BELL PEPPERS

PEACHES

STRAWBERRIES

SNAP PEAS

CUCUMBERS

APPLES

POTATOES

NECTARINES

CELERY

GRAPES
(IMPORTED)

SPINACH

CHERRY
TOMATOES

White Flour and Other Processed Ingredients

I don't keep white super-processed ingredients in the house, like white flour, sugar, or salt. They have been stripped of any nutrients they once had and are heavily processed. I basically want my food to be tampered with as little as possible. I'm not eating gluten free, but I try to avoid refined wheat products since they've been shown to spike blood sugar levels faster than some candy bars. Therefore, baking with brown rice, spelt, and oat flour instead of white flour is a better option. We keep a ton of brown rice and quinoa pasta in the house to satisfy pasta cravings. Also, I've learned over the years that certain sweeteners in moderation aren't bad for you, but I still do not use granulated sugar at all. You can satisfy that sweet craving in healthier ways—I cook with maple syrup, which is loaded with antioxidants. I also use coconut sugar, which is a great replacement for white or brown sugar.

EASY INGREDIENT SWAPS

There are lots of options these days for alternatives to white processed ingredients. Note that you can't always swap these out one for one, so taste as you go or check cookbooks for more information.

INSTEAD OF THIS:	USE THIS:
white flour	spelt, brown rice, or oat flour
white sugar	coconut sugar (swap for the exact amount)
white table salt	pink Himalayan salt or Celtic sea salt
agave	maple syrup
canola and safflower oils	ghee or coconut or olive oils

SUPPLEMENTS

I'm lucky to have a knowledgeable, integrative doctor who introduced me to many great natural supplements. It can be tough otherwise; some supplements include additives that I stay away from. I don't take anything prescription unless I absolutely have to, but there are a few supplements that I take most days.

For instance, after living in Chicago for a year, I was feeling run down, and tests showed my **VITAMIN D** levels were low. Since we get vitamin D mostly from exposure to the sun, my low D levels made sense—Chicago isn't exactly sunny Southern California! Now every day in winter, I take a vitamin D supplement (with vitamin K2 in it, which helps direct calcium into the bones and may have antiaging benefits). Your body turns vitamin D into a hormone, and its absence can be responsible for low energy, among other things. It's essential for bone health and proper functioning of the immune system. If you're feeling run down, ask your doctor to check your level.

I regularly take **FISH OIL**, whether it be in pill form or a liquid dose. I try to get some in every day. It's loaded with omega-3 fatty acids, which help reduce inflammation and are great for skin and hair.

MAGNESIUM is another beneficial supplement I take daily. A mineral that is present in relatively large amounts in the body, magnesium is fundamental to more than 300 chemical reactions that keep the body working properly, including the detoxification process, which helps eliminate damage from environmental chemicals, heavy metals, and other toxins. I've noticed that when I take magnesium close to bedtime, I sleep like a baby—which is saying a lot, because once I had kids, my good sleep habits nose-dived. Look for products other than magnesium oxide, which has more of a laxative effect and is less absorbable.

PROBIOTICS are the good bacteria we need for a healthy gut; they are incredibly beneficial and are taken by everyone in my house, including my little ones. I take one pill a day, plus I eat fermented food, which also includes probiotics. If you have to take an antibiotic, it's important to follow up the round with one probiotic every day for at least a month to replenish the good bacteria in the gut; that's because antibiotics kill all bacteria, even the good.

Finally, I take a **MULTIVITAMIN** once or twice a day (depending on what I'm eating). I eat a well-balanced diet and try to get most of my vitamins from food, so my doctor doesn't worry if I don't get in two multis a day.

Home Remedies

My family and friends used to think I was nuts for giving them oil when they had a headache or were getting sick, but after trying my remedies and having them work, now everyone is convinced!

▶ For headaches, I put peppermint oil on my temples and the back of my neck.

▶ To help fight off colds, I drink oil of oregano drops mixed in 1 or 2 ounces apple cider vinegar. It's gross, but definitely works!

▶ I put lavender oil on my feet (it absorbs through the skin quickly) and on my pillow at night when I'm traveling to help me sleep.

▶ When I know I'm going to have a couple of cocktails, I'll take two charcoal pills to reduce my hangover by a third.

▶ For a sore throat, I drink tea with lemon and manuka honey. Manuka honey has antibacterial properties and is also great on your face as a gentle exfoliant and helps acne-prone skin.

"CHEATING"

With all of that said, always watching what I eat is difficult. I cannot do it every day of the year. I'm still human! But instead of having a "cheat" day, I aim more to stay on track 80 percent of the time, and the other 20 percent I eat whatever I want and don't think twice about it. Homemade cookies, brown rice pasta, and goat cheese all apply to the 80 percent—it's everyday food that I feel good about eating. Raw nuts are a big staple in my house. I even make homemade almond milk. I eat a ton of good fats like avocados with olive oil and pink Himalayan salt; if I was hung up on calories or fat, that combination alone would be far beyond what was "acceptable" for a snack. But simply put, I believe my body can function at its highest potential when I nourish it and feed it great food.

> I aim to stay on track 80 percent of the time, and the other 20 percent I eat whatever I want.

It's the food that is possibly loaded with antibiotics and white sugar that falls into the other 20 percent. These situations usually happen when eating out or on vacation. Those times, I will eat white bread with butter (not grass-fed or organic), chicken fingers (who knows where that chicken is coming from!), non-grass-fed burgers, and pasta dishes made with white flour without hesitation. You'll never see me eating a bag of Doritos or high-fructose candy or anything processed to that degree—those types of snacks aren't real food. Even when splurging, I still only eat actual food. But 20 percent of the time, I let my rules bend so that going out to eat is enjoyable. It's empowering to have the self-control to eat these things occasionally, then the next day get back on track. I try not to torment myself too much if this 20 percent food occasionally includes small or trace amounts of added chemicals here and there. They are very hard to avoid sometimes. It's the year-after-year effect—when those chemicals compound—that feels the most dangerous to me, so I believe cutting down overall makes a huge difference. I do my very best and try not to obsess over the exceptions. In short, everything in moderation has proven itself to me. I finally feel at peace with food.

Food for the Plane

Sometimes it feels like I live on airplanes, flying back and forth from L.A., Chicago, New York, and Nashville. But you will never see me eating food from an airplane or an airport. I always bring plenty of snacks and either a salad or sandwich. This is why planning ahead is so important to stay on track, even while away from home. Here are a few of my favorite go-tos for no-fuss traveling food.

- ▶ Apple with to-go almond butter packets

- ▶ Hummus and avocado sandwich

- ▶ Homemade trail mix (a combination of almonds, cashews, walnuts, chocolate-covered goji berries, and dried cranberries is my fave)

- ▶ Oat Balls (see page 222)

- ▶ Homemade Almond Butter Sugar Cookies (see page 225)

- ▶ Healthy energy bars (I like to make my own chewy granola bars, but I also like Larabars and Amazing Grass bars. These are easy to throw in a resealable plastic bag, and they take up hardly any room.)

I've even brought leftovers like chicken with veggies or a burger on planes. Just make sure you have room in your suitcase for the container on the return flight—we use glass containers, so there's no way I'm throwing those out!

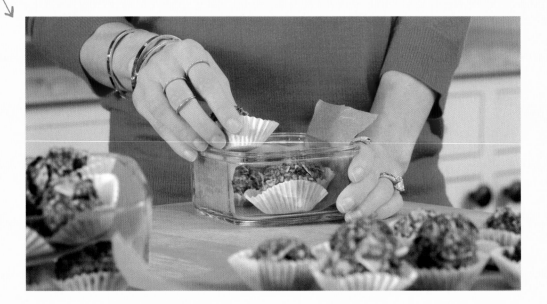

FOOD YOU'LL ALWAYS FIND IN MY HOUSE

There are certain items my family can't live without. If we have junk around, we eat it, so I strive to keep good, nutritious food in the house for quick snacks and meals or for when I haven't had time for a grocery store run. A rule I live by is to always make a colorful plate for every meal, or at least try to!

▶ **GRASS-FED GROUND BEEF**. It contains more omega-3s, more CLA (conjugated linoleic acid—associated with reduced body fat and other potential health benefits), more vitamin E, more beta-carotene, and more micronutrients (potassium, iron, zinc, phosphorus).

▶ **WILD-CAUGHT SALMON**. Wild fish are healthier because they eat sea vegetables and other fish, and naturally contain more omega-3 fatty acids. I don't eat farm-raised fish, which eat grain or corn feed or processed pellets made from small fish like anchovies and sardines, very different from the way fish eat in their natural habitat.

▶ **ORGANIC CHICKEN BREASTS AND/OR CHICKEN THIGHS**

▶ **BACON MADE WITHOUT NITRATES OR NITRITES**. All of us could eat bacon literally every single day.

▶ **APPLES AND BERRIES**. My boys love both. Jax will eat an entire carton of raspberries in one sitting!

▶ **AVOCADOS**

▶ **AT LEAST FOUR DIFFERENT KINDS OF ORGANIC GREEN VEGGIES** (often asparagus, spinach, broccoli, and especially zucchini—we all love it)

▶ **FERMENTED FOOD**. Jalapeño sauerkraut is my new obsession, but I also like garlic sauerkraut and fermented pickles.

▶ **ORGANIC EGGS**. Hard-cooked eggs are a great, easy snack or quick morning breakfast. I do a few at a time and keep them in the fridge.

▶ **RAW GOAT'S MILK CHEDDAR CHEESE**. I could, and sometimes do, eat this every day!

▶ **HOMEMADE ALMOND MILK**

▶ **HOMEMADE SPINACH HUMMUS**. A batch of this every week means easy lunches and snacks.

▶ **SPROUTED BREAD**

▶ **QUINOA**

▶ **BROWN RICE PASTA**

▶ **ROLLED OATS**

▶ **NUTS**

▶ **ALMOND BUTTER AND NATURAL PEANUT BUTTER**. Ingredients should consist only of almonds/peanuts and maybe a little salt.

▶ **REAL MAPLE SYRUP**

▶ **COCONUT OIL, OLIVE OIL**

▶ **APPLE CIDER VINEGAR**. This does everything: eases tummy troubles, gets rid of colds, soothes sore throats, and boosts energy.

▶ **ALOE JUICE**. A shot keeps your digestive system moving, if ya know what I mean!

▶ **MACA POWDER** (from a plant grown in central Peru known to boost energy, help balance hormones, and boost the immune system). I use this in smoothies and lattes (see the Maca Turmeric Latte recipe on page 206).

▶ **CHIA SEEDS**

▶ **DARK CHOCOLATE**

▶ **SOME SORT OF HOMEMADE SWEET,** usually Almond Butter Sugar Cookies (see the recipe on page 225) or brownies

▶ **HOT SAUCE!!** We can't have enough around. We like Sriracha and Cholula on just about everything, even though there are a few ingredients I'm not thrilled about. I just love them too much to say no!

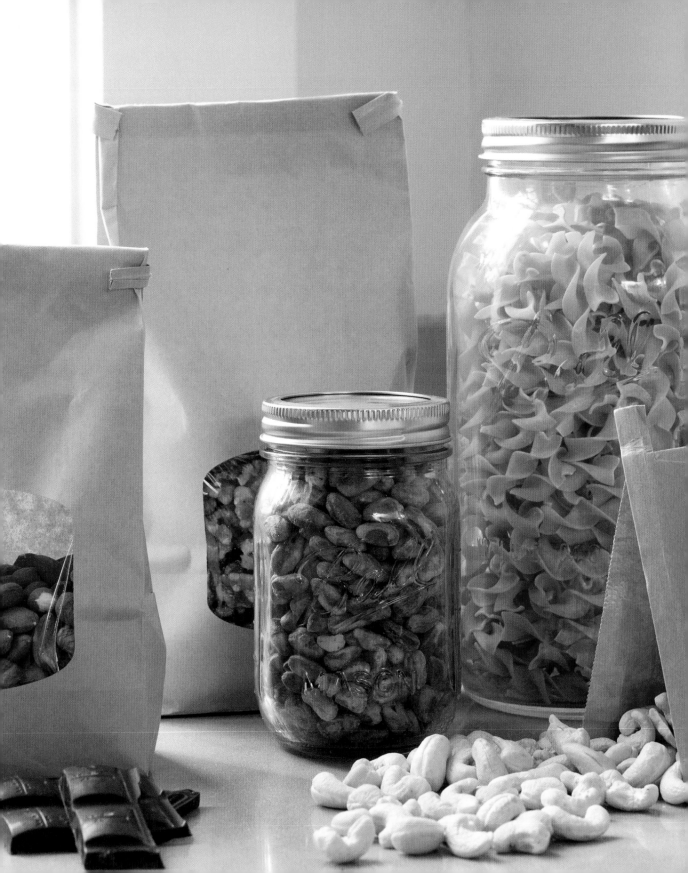

FOOD YOU'LL NEVER FIND IN MY HOUSE

I don't keep any of the following items in my house. While I occasionally eat white flour and sugar at a restaurant or on vacation, I won't eat them at home, ever. For example, as much as I love to cook, I will not keep ingredients to make biscuits and gravy (cow's milk and white flour) around the house. Jay would be in heaven, and it is something we'll eat for breakfast out, once in a blue moon, but I won't buy the stuff to make them so that we're not tempted every weekend.

▶ **SUGARY CEREAL**

▶ **DORITOS** (or any other highly processed chip)

▶ **SPORTS DRINKS**

▶ **CORN, UNLESS IT'S ORGANIC**

▶ **OREOS** (or any other processed cookie)

▶ **SODA**

▶ **CONVENTIONAL MILK** (nonorganic is loaded with hormones and antibiotics, but because of my casein allergy, I don't buy organic either)

▶ **WHITE FLOUR**

▶ **WHITE SUGAR**

▶ **ANY LOW-FAT, LOW-CALORIE DIET FOOD**

▶ **TOFU** (It freaks me out, to be completely honest! I'm weirded out by fake meats too, since they're just big blocks of soy usually. I avoid soy for the most part since it messes with estrogen and is usually GMO.)

▶ **VEGAN CHEESE** (Since it's not real cheese, it doesn't really do it for me.)

▶ **GLUTEN-FREE PRODUCTS** (no good nutrition, just empty carbs, plus more expensive)

AMATEUR CHEF

I started cooking when Camden was born because all he did was sleep and I needed something productive and creative to do. Like I said earlier, I was living in a new city and my husband was knee-deep in the football season, so I had a lot of alone time. Because I've always loved food and envisioned myself cooking for my family every night, I decided to start cooking on my own and see what happened. The most I could do at the time was make a salad or a boxed brownie mix, which says something about how I used to eat! After some failed attempts, like homemade ravioli (what was I thinking making those for my second meal ever?!), things started to click pretty quickly. And I *loved* it.

I found cooking to be therapeutic and a nice break from the day-to-day stresses. It had an added bonus: I was sure about what I was feeding my family, instead of buying something at the store and hoping it was good for us. I liked taking my family's health into my own hands.

> I honestly believe you can do almost anything for your personal health through food. Food can be medicinal, preventive, you name it.

In addition to learning the benefits of healthy eating and cooking for my own body, I've now seen what a good diet can do for others' bodies as well. Jay has type 1 diabetes, and his numbers have drastically changed since he adopted this healthy lifestyle. His insulin use is down, and he's off of his blood pressure medication. And he looks the best he ever has: His weight is ideal and his skin is clear. I really believe that my family's infrequency of getting sick is due to our diet. I honestly believe you can do almost anything for your personal health through food. Food can be medicinal, preventive, you name it. This is why cooking for my family gives me power and makes me feel good. My mom once said that she shows her love through cooking for people, and I'm starting to feel as though I do that in some ways too.

Camden loves to sit on the counter and be my little helper. He's usually my taste tester more than anything, but it's fun that he loves the process. Jay isn't too bad of a cook himself. He takes over the kitchen some nights, letting me relax, and I love it. I am so glad that dinner is something everyone in my family is involved with.

Now I cook most nights and cherish dinnertime. I grew up with my family gathered at the dinner table every night, and that's a tradition I continue with my children. It's a time to connect and catch up on the day and just be together as a family without outside distractions. I love sitting down on the couch Sunday night with cookbooks or written ideas from the week in hand and figuring out the menu for the days ahead. I can usually plan for 4 or 5 days and get all my shopping done in one trip. I'm a list girl (type A!), so I venture to the store with a massive list and check things off as I go.

Ideas for Easy, Healthy Breakfasts

Breakfasts are important. This first meal sets the tone for the entire day. I never skip breakfast. If I'm going to the gym early, I'll just whip up a smoothie, otherwise I eat a fairly decent-size meal.

- ▶ **FRIED EGG** with quinoa, spinach, and bacon

- ▶ **SCRAMBLED EGGS** in a sprouted tortilla with raw goat's milk Cheddar cheese and salsa

- ▶ **EGG SANDWICH:** two fried eggs with organic mayo and hot sauce between two pieces of sprouted bread

- ▶ **GREEN BANANA MUFFINS** (see the recipe on page 205)

- ▶ A **SMOOTHIE** with spinach or kale thrown in for added greens

- ▶ **OVERNIGHT CHIA-OAT CUPS** (see the recipe on page 202) topped with berries, chocolate chips, shaved coconut, and almonds...there are endless options

- ▶ **OATMEAL** (rolled oats) with ground flaxseeds, 1 teaspoon coconut oil, and maple syrup

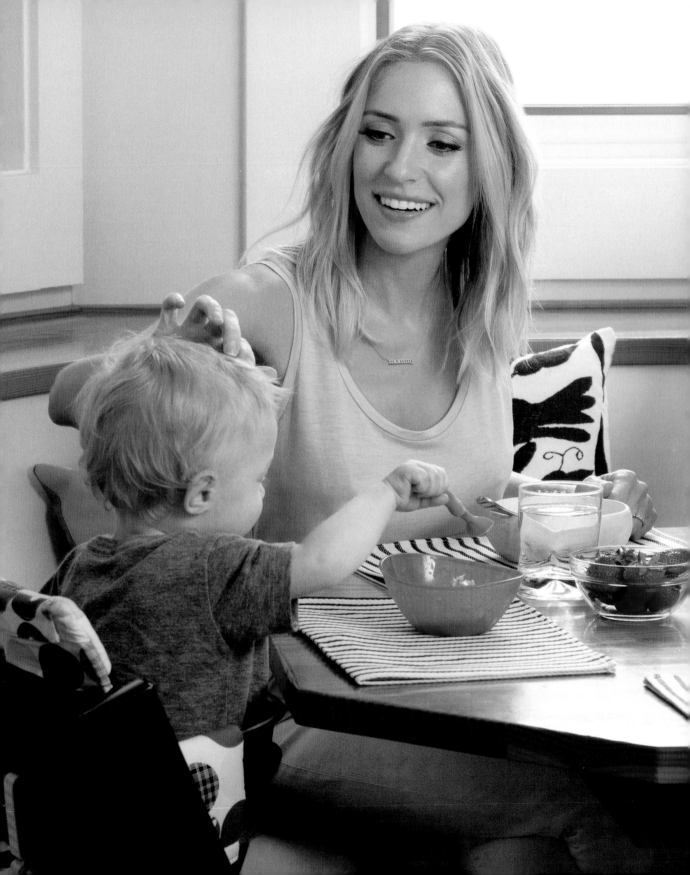

Ideas for Quick Lunches

For me, lunches are usually painless, since midday meals made with leftovers are a go-to in my house. But if I have the time, I'll whip something up while Cam is at school.

▶ **SALAD WITH CANNED TUNA OR CHICKPEAS** and lots of raw or cooked leftover veggies. I usually make my own salad dressings, but occasionally I use store-bought ones if the ingredients are okay.

▶ **HUMMUS AND AVOCADO WRAP** with tomato, lettuce, olive oil, and balsamic vinegar

▶ **BROCCOLI SALAD WITH AVOCADO MAYO** (see the recipe on page 220)

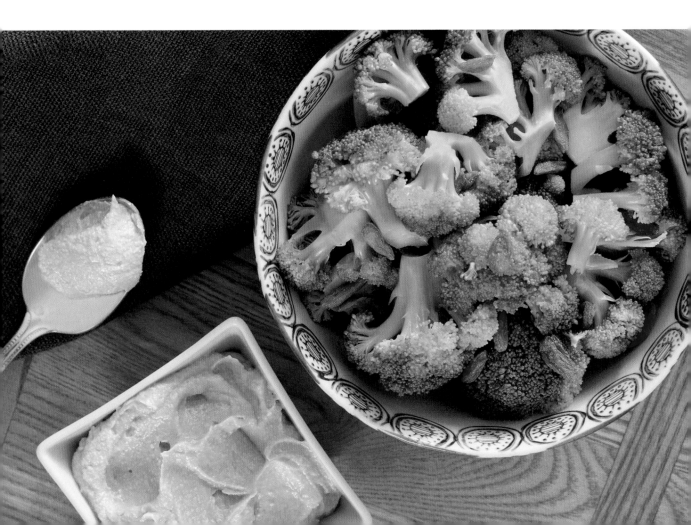

- **CHERRY-PISTACHIO QUINOA** (see the recipe on page 215). This keeps well in the fridge, so I like to make a big batch early in the week.

- I like slow roasting a chicken all day Sunday (I throw a whole chicken in a Dutch oven with coconut oil, salt, and pepper—see the recipe on page 211) and using that meat for **SANDWICHES** and **WRAPS** that week. I usually put mayo, lettuce, tomato, chicken, a couple slices of raw goat's milk Cheddar cheese, and sometimes a few drops of hot sauce on a sprouted tortilla or sprouted bread.

- I could eat **SOUP** year-round. Doesn't matter if it's 80 degrees outside, I'll eat it! I love any kind of veggie soup because you get a ton of greens, and soup is comforting, even without all the heavy cream. Plus, you can soak cashews in water, then puree them to add a little dairy-free creamy texture to tomato or asparagus soup.

Dinners for When You Are Alone with the Kids

When you are solo with the little ones, getting dinner ready can be a challenge. I always plan ahead to make it as easy as possible.

- **HEALTHY ENCHILADAS** made with raw goat's milk Cheddar cheese and a side salad or cut-up bell peppers. I make pumpkin cupcakes for a yummy dessert.

- Mix grass-fed beef with salt, pepper, garlic, and onion to make **BUNLESS BURGERS**. Sauté zucchini in olive oil and top with garlic salt. Whole sweet potatoes are easy to throw in the oven and are loved by everyone in my house for a side.

- **GRASS-FED GROUND BEEF IN TOMATO SAUCE OVER BROWN RICE SPAGHETTI**. (I make my own sauce when I make homemade meatballs and freeze leftovers, but I also love Rao's and Amy's store-bought sauces.) I usually just cut up some cucumbers for the boys and me as a serving of green veggie.

- **CHICKEN TACOS:** chicken thighs prepared in the slow cooker, put into a brown rice tortilla, and topped with guacamole, salsa, raw goat's milk Cheddar cheese, beans, and shredded lettuce. I like chicken thighs because they taste better and don't dry out. I'm obsessed with my slow cooker, since you throw everything in and forget about it—just about as easy as you can get!

▶ **BREAKFAST FOR DINNER** is a go-to when I haven't been to the store. Cashew Pancakes (see the recipe on page 201) are full of protein and taste great. We top ours with grass-fed butter and plenty of maple syrup. Scrambled eggs usually accompany the pancakes as well.

Date Dinners for You and Hubby

Jay and I make a conscious effort to have regular date nights. Sometimes staying home and opening a bottle of wine are all we have the energy for, and they usually end up being the best nights. To start, we both love cheese, so a plate with goat's and sheep's milk cheeses and store-bought flaxseed crackers is usually on the counter while I prepare dinner. To end, homemade brownies are always welcome. Dim the lights, put on some mellow music, and wear comfy clothes.

▶ **MISO SALMON** (see the recipe on page 208) and **SWEET MISO BRUSSELS SPROUTS** (see the recipe on page 214) This salmon is one of our favorites. I could eat this miso dressing on everything!

▶ One of Jay's favorite meals is **LEEK AND BEAN STEW WITH CHICKEN**. It's a great comfort dish when it's cold outside. I try to make it frequently, since I know how much he loves it.

▶ **STEAK WITH BUTTERY MUSHROOMS AND CAULIFLOWER "MASHED POTATOES."** This was one of the first meals I ever made for Jay (although I made regular mashed potatoes), so it brings us back to the early days of our relationship. I had no clue what I was doing in the kitchen, so I called my mom and she told me to make this meal. A man favorite!

Dinners to Impress the In-laws (Or Your Own Parents)

We love having both of our families over. Luckily, they're close by, so we see them often. I love my mother-in-law because she is easygoing and would be happy eating just a big salad for dinner if that's all we offered. She takes the pressure off completely!

▶ **STUFFED JALAPEÑO PEPPERS WITH CHICKEN SAUSAGE, CHEESE, AND SPICES** for an appetizer, followed by beer-can chicken (Jay grills a whole chicken with a half-full beer can shoved inside the body—delicious!) and buttery green beans or broccoli sprinkled with a little garlic salt.

▶ **HOMEMADE MEATBALLS AND BROWN RICE SPAGHETTI,** with a salad on the side—it's a family recipe.

▶ **DAIRY-FREE MUSHROOM–PEA RISOTTO** (see the recipe on page 213) with bison tenderloin. End with sea salt "Caramel" Bites (see the recipe on page 221).

Dinners with the Girls

When friends come to visit from out of town, our Saturday cooking nights are a blast. We usually have a big platter of veggies with homemade ranch dip to snack on while we cook dinner. We open a bottle of organic wine, and everyone helps out.

▶ **SLOW-ROASTED CHICKEN WITH CHIPOTLE SAUCE** (see the recipe on page 211). We make skinny margaritas (tequila with lime juice and maple syrup) and nibble on tortilla chips (non-GMO and without scary chemicals) with homemade guacamole and salsa.

▶ **STIR-FRY WITH BROWN RICE, TONS OF VEGGIES, AND SHRIMP.** We end with Chocolate Hemp Pudding (see the recipe on page 226)—because we all love chocolate.

▶ Jay makes us dinner periodically—everything from **GRILLED FISH AND VEGGIES** to a unique-to-Jay favorite: a big platter of spaghetti squash topped with sausage and zucchini, yellow squash, mushrooms, and green peppers mixed with pizza sauce. Sounds weird, but it's amazing!

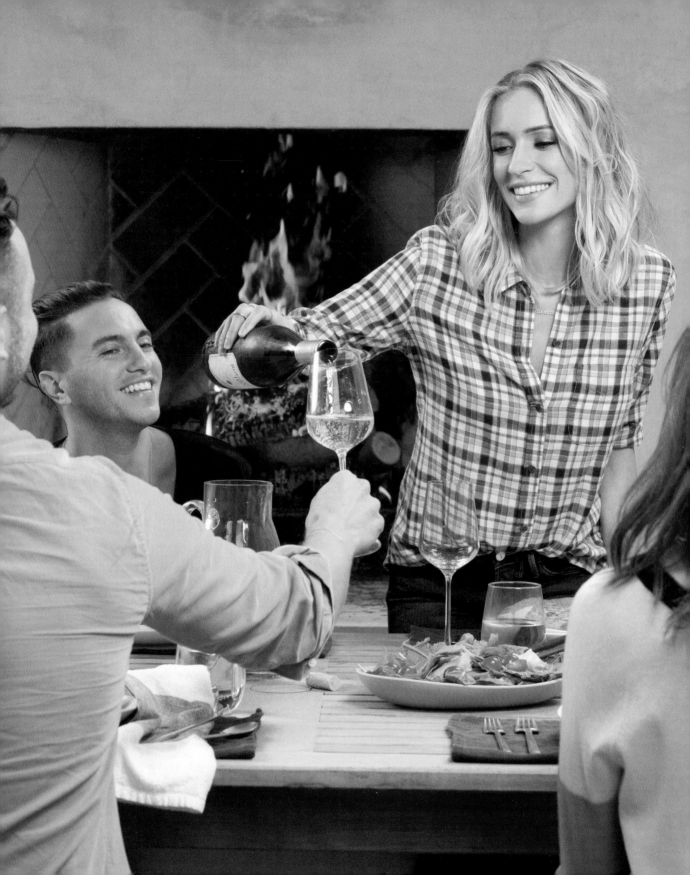

Dinner Parties

There's nothing I love more than having a few friends over for a fun dinner party. I go all out—I've even made ice-cream sandwiches—and spend the whole day prepping in the kitchen. I always have fresh flowers and candles burning. When we're in Nashville, we open the doors and Jay mans the grill while everyone catches up around the pool. We're laid-back; I don't stress about everyone having the same kind of glass—if some people have plastic cups and others wineglasses (we always serve organic wine), that's fine by me! It's all about getting the people we love together, whether it be family or close friends, and having some fun.

▶ **BUFFALO MOZZARELLA WITH TOMATOES AND KALE PESTO,** homemade artichoke dip with store-bought flaxseed crackers (or other "clean" crackers), beef or bison tenderloin, buttery green beans, Cauliflower "Potato" Salad (see the recipe on page 218), and homemade chocolate chip cookies.

▶ **DEVILED EGGS** are one of my favorite appetizers. The mayo I use is made with organic eggs, and every time I make deviled eggs, I could eat about 12! Cheeseless Queso Dip (it's cashews; see the recipe on page 217) is another crowd favorite. You don't have to tell your guests it's not real queso (unless they have nut allergies!)—they will never know. Trust me! Quinoa with black beans, tomatoes, and scallions is great for a big group. I serve it with Brussels sprouts (roasted with honey, thyme, lemon, and olive oil) and grilled chicken thighs and veggies. "Caramel" Bites (see the recipe on page 221) are for dessert.

▶ **BACON-WRAPPED BUTTERNUT SQUASH** (always a hit and super-easy), homemade flatbread with goat's cheese and pears (I use whole wheat flour for this), sautéed scallops over wilted spinach, cauliflower "mashed potatoes," and chocolate-covered strawberries.

Balancing It All

Food has a huge impact on my overall wellness. Not only is my skin glowing, but I feel great and don't have to worry about dieting. I'm able to enjoy life and not obsess about how many calories I consume in one day. When I take care of my body the majority of the time, I'm able to eat things I usually wouldn't when I have the urge. Occasionally not caring if something is genetically modified and eating things I don't normally consume (white bread and sugar) actually keep me on track. I don't feel like I'm missing out on anything, and it makes me appreciate good, quality food. Plus, I've learned that after a big, fattening meal with empty calories, I feel run down, tired, and lazy. It spurs me to get back to the great way I normally feel when I eat nutritious food.

Taking my health and that of my family into my own hands has been empowering—it's super-gratifying to see the people around me feel the best they ever have. I want to live long enough to see my babies grow and start families of their own, and I know that through eating real food, I will. I recommend taking charge of your own diet and health and eating only real food. You'll feel and look the best you can.

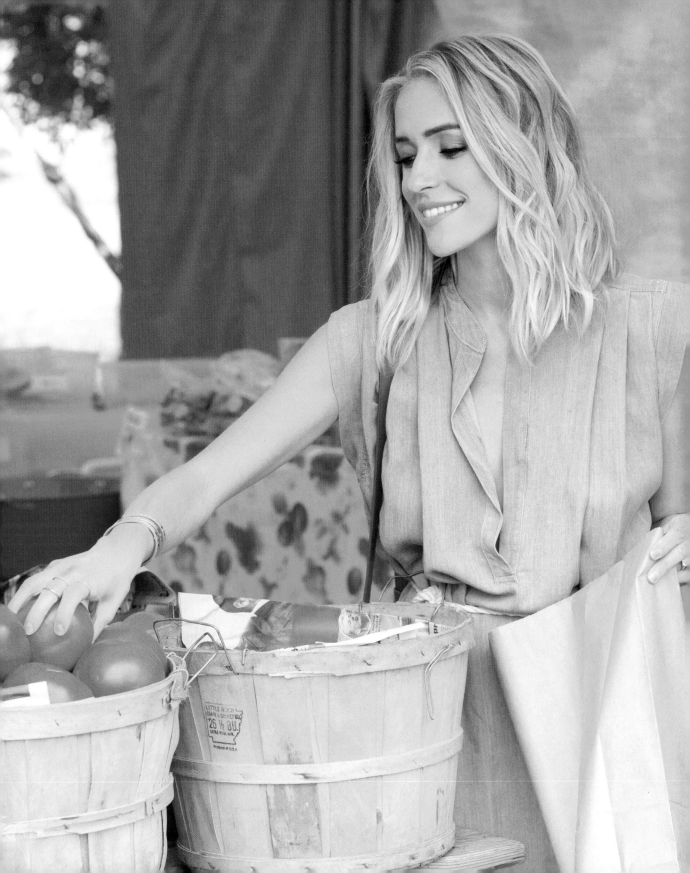

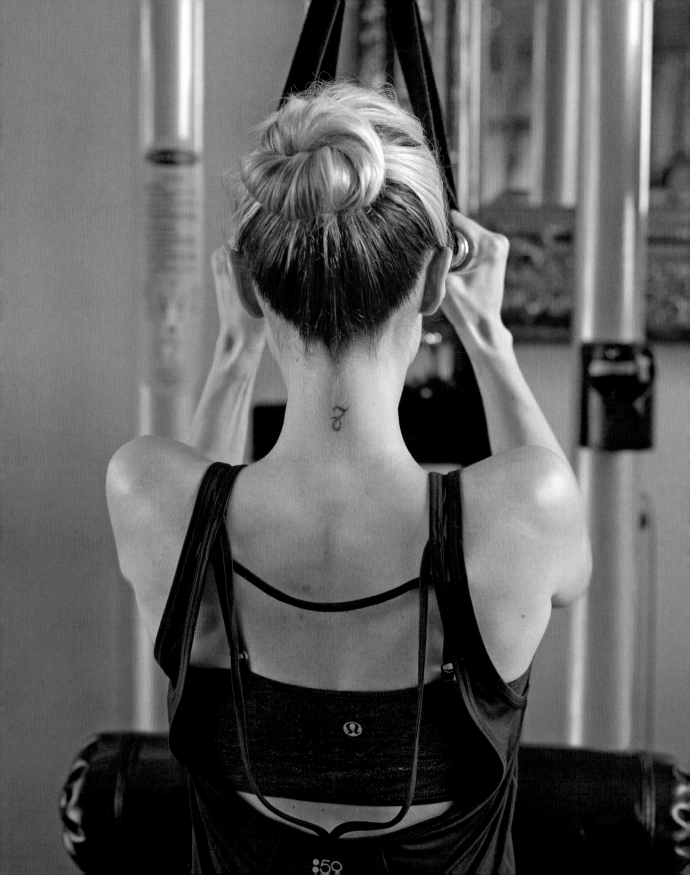

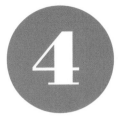
Work It Out

IN MY EARLY TWENTIES, I HAD A MENTALLY EXHAUSTING relationship with working out. I was never comfortable and happy in my own skin and always wanted to lose weight. It was a constant battle of not being thin enough, so I would obsess over going to the gym and beat myself up when I didn't work out at least four times a week. But at the same time, I was lazy and never challenged myself when I did make it to the gym. I loved the elliptical machine and walking uphill on the treadmill because I could take it as slow as I wanted. Once 30 minutes was through, I was out the door. I thought because I put in the time (even though 30 minutes likely wasn't enough anyway), I would magically get in shape. Back then, all I cared about was the number on the scale, so cardio was my best friend—or so I assumed. I didn't think about building muscle to help burn fat or changing up my workouts to keep my body guessing. I went through spurts of working out with a trainer but never committed long term. Overall, I was focused on the wrong thing. I was looking for a quick fix, an easy way to get particular results. I didn't realize there is no such thing.

After I had children, everything changed. Going through three pregnancies and becoming a mother made me respect my body so much for everything it went through. Because of that, I became more comfortable with the body I had and worried less about it being "ideal." But another strange thing happened: After kids, I got too thin. While it might seem like being "too thin" would suddenly resolve all my weight conflicts, it instead made me think differently about my body and its overall health. After the extreme changes your body goes through when pregnant, all I wanted postpregnancy was to be a normal weight and as healthy as I could for myself and my family. Being too thin didn't work for me—besides the simple fact that I just didn't like the way my body looked, my babies relied on me to be above a certain weight and healthy since I was breastfeeding and supplying their milk (even though part of the reason I was burning so many calories was because of breastfeeding!). Instead of trying everything to lose weight, now I had to work hard at keeping muscle on and maintaining a healthy number on the scale. I haven't done cardio since before I had kids because I get too thin. Instead, I usually weight train three times a week (if I go more than a week without lifting weights, I notice my muscle vanishing) and do Pilates twice a week to strengthen my core, since that's my problem area.

My perspective on exercise and its relation to body image changed: I now see working out as an opportunity to improve my overall health and maintain a healthy weight, not as a time to try to change my body to be something else. This feels like a more centered and reasonable approach no matter what size my body

> I now see working out as an opportunity to improve my overall health and maintain a healthy weight, not as a time to try to change my body to be something else.

is. Further, with this changed mind-set, I realized I actually *liked* the act of working out. It gave me something positive to work toward and was a stress-relieving time I could take just for me.

WHY I LOVE WORKING OUT

When I'm consistent with my workouts, I have more energy and I'm a happier person. I get my frustration out at the gym and always leave in a great mood. If I'm feeling stressed or tired, working out makes me forget what I was upset about and zaps my lethargic butt in gear. If I'm gonna be there at all, I might as well get the most out of it, so my workouts are a time when I push myself! I've realized that I need the physical *and* mental challenge.

Today, I feel the strongest I ever have, and I'm happy to say I'm finally comfortable in my own skin. Of course, there are little things that bug me, just like everyone else, but overall I'm at peace with my body. I used to feel like I was at war with my body, but exercising now makes me feel like I'm working *with* it to help myself be a better person physically and mentally. I make a conscious effort to focus on what I like about my body instead of what I wish I had. Everyone's body is different, and now I embrace that instead of trying to change something I have little control over. I used to get hung up on wanting bigger hips, for example, but no matter how much weight I gain, I will never have curvy hips. And I'm okay with that.

All Ready for the Gym

Getting prepared to work out is supersimple. I don't wear any makeup, I remove my rings and any other jewelry (with the exception of a small necklace), and I pull my hair back. I arrive at the gym dressed and ready to go. I keep my clothes basic: leggings to my shin or ankle, a sports bra, and a tank top or T-shirt. It's fun to add a pop of color, so I wear bright shoes, anything from hot pink to teal.

The Power of Keeping Track

There are a few ways I make working out fulfilling for myself. I love setting mini goals, whether the goal is lifting a certain amount of weight after a couple of weeks or gaining a pound. Having goals to work toward (and changing them up) keeps my mind engaged so I don't get bored. It's also a great feeling reaching whatever I was trying to accomplish.

To help, I write everything down: what the exercise is, how much weight I use, how many reps, and the date. I strive to increase the weight or at least stay the same. I never go down in weight. Writing it out reminds me of where I am and encourages me to track my progress. These records are something I can look back on and be proud of. (Usually! Bad gym days happen too.) Check out the charts on pages 127 and 132 for some examples.

Nourishing Your Body Before and After Working Out

I've learned from my trainer that when weight training and trying to gain weight, it's crucial to consume some protein within 30 minutes of working out. I make sure to do this since I'm constantly trying to maintain or gain muscle. My trainer makes me a protein shake directly after I finish my session, and a few nights a week before bed I drink a different protein shake I prepare at home. Protein is crucial for building muscle and burning fat. Even if you aren't trying to gain weight, protein is still important. The more muscle mass you have, the more fat you can burn.

No matter what your exercise goal, staying hydrated is incredibly important. I'm constantly drinking water; I have a water bottle with me wherever I go. While working out, I mix branched-chain amino acids in my water for extra protein. I down almost an entire large bottle (32 ounces) of H_2O during each workout, and I try to drink two more bottles throughout the day. The only downside of being super-hydrated is that you pee every 2 seconds (or so it seems), but the health benefits make it worth it!

PRE/POSTWORKOUT SNACKS

After I weight train, I always drink a protein shake and I usually eat a snack or lunch within 30 minutes as well. If I do Pilates, I won't have a protein shake, but I make sure to eat something within the hour. Working out gives me a huge appetite!

- Protein shake
- Oat Balls (see the recipe on page 222)—easy to put in a resealable plastic bag and bring wherever you go

- Apple with almond butter
- Trail mix

THE WORKOUTS

I have a tendency to get bored when it comes to working out—and being bored is not conducive to scheduling regular exercise sessions. Back in high school, I did Bikram yoga a few times a week and got burnt out quickly since it's the exact same thing. Every. Single. Time. Today, I'm always changing up exercise. I do three different workouts each week, repeating for 4 weeks, then do completely different ones for the next 4 weeks, and so on. Not only does this keep my mind from getting bored, but it keeps my muscles guessing as well. When you change up your workouts, your body never gets complacent and works at its highest potential.

TIPS FROM MY TRAINER

My trainer, Mike Sorrentino, trains some of the best Chicago athletes. He has helped me put some pounds on, but he's also responsible for getting many women in tip-top shape and helping them shed weight. Mike uses a no-nonsense approach to working out that pushes you past your comfort zone. His systematic and scientific method to designing workouts has been cultivated from learning under the top strength coaches in the world. He does it all! His top tips for working out:

▶ **CONSISTENCY IS KEY.** Sticking to a weekly routine and not skipping workouts are paramount in making significant strides in your body composition goals.

▶ **KEEP WORKOUTS TO BETWEEN 45 AND 60 MINUTES.** Anything longer and your body's cortisol levels will rise dramatically. Cortisol is a stress hormone that will prevent your body from burning fat and will actually cause your body to store fat.

▶ **KEEP IT SIMPLE AND STICK TO THE BASICS.** Don't get caught up in fitness gadgets. Nothing beats using barbells, dumbbells, cables, and good old hard work.

▶ **FORM IS MORE IMPORTANT THAN EXTRA REPS.** Lift weight in a slow and controlled manner, making sure perfect form is used. By doing this, you reduce the risk of injury and ensure that the proper muscles are being targeted.

▶ **PLAN AHEAD.** Have your workout written ahead of time so that you can track your work and ensure you make progress.

Building Muscle Workout

When I strictly want to gain weight and build muscle, I do lower reps with higher weight.* Here is a sample workout.

Perform the exercises in each letter pairing back-to-back, then take a 90-second rest. Complete four sets of each pairing before moving on to the next letter pairing. The only series that is not a pairing is the D series with three different moves. Lift heavy and push yourself! The last 2 reps of each set should be very difficult. To track your progress, see page 127.

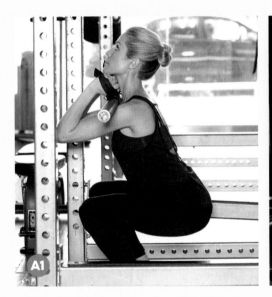

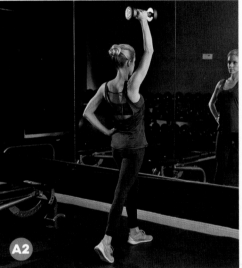

HEELS-ELEVATED FRONT SQUATS
(5–7 reps)
Elevate heels 1–2 inches. Grab bar at shoulder width, drive elbows forward, and rest bar on top of shoulders (keep as close to neck as possible). Elbows should always be as high as shoulders. To start movement, drive knees forward and lower all the way down while keeping torso upright. Then return to starting position.

SINGLE-ARM DUMBBELL SHOULDER PRESS
(standing 8–10 reps)
Hold dumbbell in neutral position starting at the shoulder. Place opposite foot forward. To start, press dumbbell straight overhead, trying to touch biceps to ear. Then lower back to starting position.

*To tailor this workout to be more fat-burning, you can use lower weight and higher reps, or you can add some cardio to burn more calories. Or just go to the Burning Calories Workout on page 130!

Building Muscle Workout (continued)

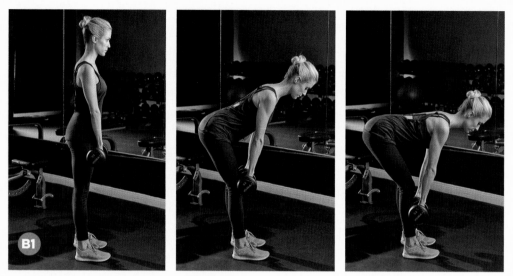

DUMBBELL ROMANIAN DEADLIFT (RDL)
(8–10 reps)

Stand with feet just inside shoulder width. Bend knees 5 degrees just outside of lockout. Hinge over at waist, keeping dumbbells touching thighs the whole time. Lower until moderate stretch is felt in hamstrings while keeping back flat. Return to starting position and push hips through by squeezing glutes to finish.

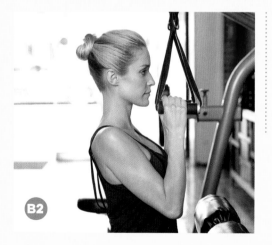

CABLE PULLDOWN
(8–10 reps)

Hold handles in a neutral position (palms facing each other) and pinch shoulder blades down and back. Pull handles straight down to shoulder and return to starting position.

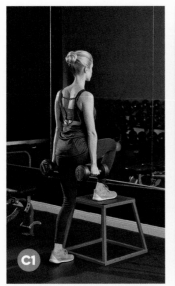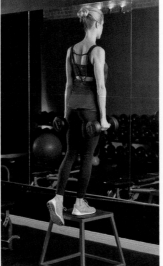

STEP-UPS KNEE HIGH
(10 reps each leg)

Start with foot on knee-high box. Load weight on working leg (front foot), drive knee over toe while keeping heel down, and push straight up without using other leg to cheat. At top, squeeze glute, then lower back to starting position. Complete all reps on one leg, then switch.

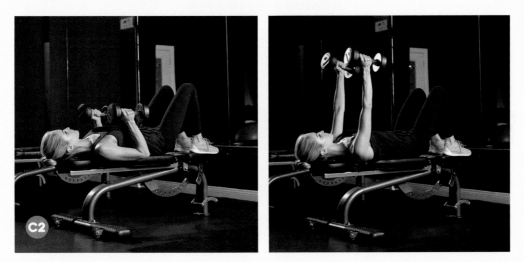

FLAT DUMBBELL CHEST PRESS
(8–10 reps)

Lie flat on bench; if back is too arched due to bench height, then feet can go on bench as well. Start with dumbbells in neutral position. Push straight up without touching dumbbells at top. As you lower dumbbells, pinch shoulder blades together while having the elbows track out at a 45-degree angle.

Building Muscle Workout *(continued)*

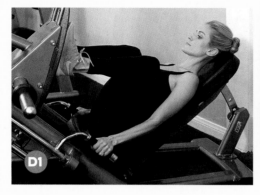

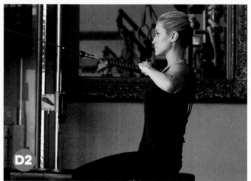

CLOSE STANCE LEG PRESS— FEET 4–6 INCHES APART

(10–12 reps)

Start with feet 4–6 inches apart, toes slightly pointed out. Lower weight as far down as possible, letting knees track out slightly. To return to starting position, push evenly through both feet without allowing heels to come off platform.

ROW TO NECK ON SEATED CABLE ROW—USE ROPE

(10–12 reps)

Start by pinching shoulder blades back and down, thumbs pointed down, and palms facing out. Pull rope straight to chin level, keeping elbows same height as shoulders. Return to starting position.

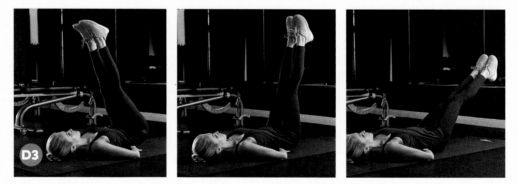

LYING LEG LOWERING ON FLOOR

(12–15 reps)

Lie flat on back, placing hands palms down under lumbar spine (not tailbone). Start with feet straight up in the air, toes pointing to each other. Push lower back into hands and lower legs until all pressure of low back is off hands. Then return to starting position.

Building Muscle Workout Chart

			DATE:		DATE:		DATE:		DATE:		DATE:	
			Weight	Reps	Weight	Reps	Weight	Reps	Weight	Reps	Weight	Reps
A1	HEELS-ELEVATED FRONT SQUATS Reps: 5–7	Set 1										
		Set 2										
		Set 3										
		Set 4										
A2	SINGLE-ARM DUMBBELL SHOULDER PRESS Reps: 8–10	Set 1										
		Set 2										
		Set 3										
		Set 4										
B1	DUMBBELL ROMANIAN DEADLIFT (RDL) Reps: 8–10	Set 1										
		Set 2										
		Set 3										
		Set 4										
B2	CABLE PULLDOWN Reps: 8–10	Set 1										
		Set 2										
		Set 3										
		Set 4										
C1	STEP-UPS KNEE HIGH Reps: 10 each leg	Set 1										
		Set 2										
		Set 3										
		Set 4										
C2	FLAT DUMBBELL CHEST PRESS Reps: 8–10	Set 1										
		Set 2										
		Set 3										
		Set 4										
D1	CLOSE STANCE LEG PRESS Reps: 10–12	Set 1										
		Set 2										
		Set 3										
		Set 4										
D2	ROW TO NECK ON SEATED CABLE ROW Reps: 10–12	Set 1										
		Set 2										
		Set 3										
		Set 4										
D3	LYING LEG LOWERING ON FLOOR Reps: 12–15	Set 1										
		Set 2										
		Set 3										
		Set 4										

Alternative Moves for Building Muscle

You can swap any of these moves into the letter pairings in the Building Muscle Workout.

A SERIES

A1 **WIDE STANCE BACK SQUATS:** Start standing straight up with barbell on back of neck just below shoulders, feet two steps outside shoulder width with toes pointing slightly out. Drive knees forward and sit back as you lower all the way down. Keep back upright push through the heels and return to starting position.

A2 **SEATED DUMBBELL PRESS, BOTH ARMS:** Sit on bench with back unsupported, hold dumbbells in neutral position (palms facing each other) starting at the shoulder. To start press dumbbells straight overhead trying to touch biceps to ears. Then lower back to starting position.

B SERIES

B1 **LYING LEG CURL, TOES POINTED IN:** Lie stomach down on leg curl and turn toes in so that they are pointing toward each other. Curl legs up so pad makes contact with back of hamstring. Then lower to starting position.

B2 **SINGLE-ARM DUMBBELL ROW:** Kneel over side of bench by placing knee and hand of supporting arm on bench. Put opposite leg out and back so torso is flat. Grasp dumbbell from the floor and pull up so elbow touches side of body while maintaining a flat back and torso. Lower weight to starting position.

C SERIES

C1 **DROP LUNGES:** Start standing or seated. Hold dumbbells so that palms are facing in front. Curl dumbbell all the way up so biceps is touching forearm. Rotate dumbbell so palms are facing floor and lower to starting position.

C2 **ZOTTMAN CURL:** Place feet so front half of foot is on platform, lower heels toward ground until calves are in a stretched position, then flex calves so heels come as high up as possible.

D SERIES

D1 **HEELS-ELEVATED CYCLIST SQUAT OR SEATED CALF RAISE:** Elevate heels 2-4 inches, and stand with feet 4-6 inches apart. Hold dumbbells to side, drive knees forward and sit back into heels going all the way down so hamstrings touch calves. Return to starting position by driving through heels and standing up.

D2 **LYING DUMBBELL TRICEPS EXTENSION:** Stand sideways in 45-degree back extension so hip is at the top of pad. From this position, bend sideways getting a good stretch through obliques on opposite side without feet coming off platform. Then using the same obliques that was stretched return to starting position.

D3 **SIDE FLEXION:** Lie flat on back with arms fully extended and palms facing each other. Lower weight by bending from elbow so dumbbell touches shoulder. Return to starting position.

Hotel Room Workout

I'm always on the road. Sometimes I have time for only a few moves in my hotel room while I let my hair air-dry before blow-drying it. Even if this workout isn't extensive, it's better than nothing. Here are some easy moves for when you aren't at a gym.

▶ **TRICEPS DIPS** on the sofa or coffee table or dresser.

▶ **WALKING LUNGES** holding water bottles or anything else you have lying around.

▶ **SINGLE-LEG-UP LUNGES**: Put one leg on a chair and do forward lunges in place.

▶ **BRIDGE**: Lie on your back on the floor, bend your knees, and keep your feet planted on the floor, then elevate your butt in the air and squeeze it as hard as you can.

▶ **PLANK**: Hold for up to a minute. Repeat at least two times.

▶ **PUSHUPS OFF THE DRESSER OR FLOOR.** Before I started working out with my trainer, I could do literally only two real pushups, but now I can do about 15! I still sometimes do the girly ones with my knees bent; then I can get closer to 30. Start small and work your way up!

▶ **RUN THE HOTEL STAIRS** if you are feeling adventurous!

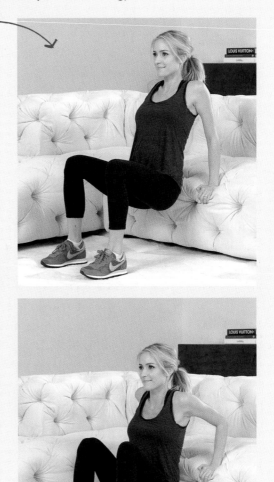

Burning Calories Workout/Crunch Time Workout

Burning calories isn't necessarily a goal of mine these days, but occasionally if I'm preparing for a photo shoot or going on vacation and won't be working out for a week, my trainer will increase the number of reps and reduce the rest periods. I typically weight train 3 days a week, but if I have a photo shoot coming up, I try to train four or five times a week. So here in the following sequence, you can knock out weight training and cardio essentially at the same time, since the pace of this workout is fast and keeps your heart rate up. This workout burns calories, tones muscle, and gets your heart pumping!

Do the five exercises ahead in a row, performing each exercise for 60 seconds and with light-to-medium weight, without any rest between them. Once all five exercises are completed, rest for 60 seconds before beginning that cycle again. Perform this sequence a total of five times. Use the chart on page 132 to track your progress.

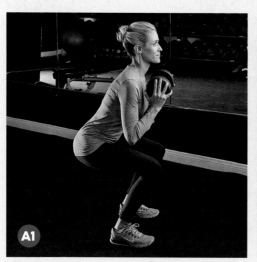

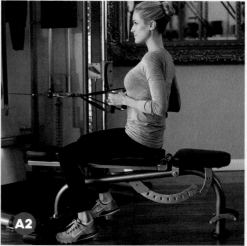

SQUATS WITH DUMBBELLS
Start standing straight up, feet just outside shoulder width with toes pointing slightly out. Hold dumbbells below chin. Drive knees forward and sit back as you lower all the way down. Keep back upright, push through heels, and return to starting position.

SEATED ROW
Start with torso upright. Grab handles in neutral position (palms facing each other), while keeping arms straight. Pinch shoulder blades back and down. Pull handles straight back, allowing the forearms to touch side of body. Lower weight on the same path and return to starting position.

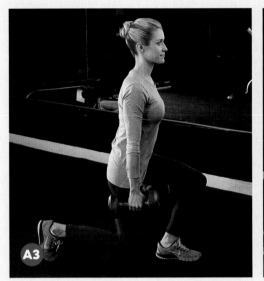

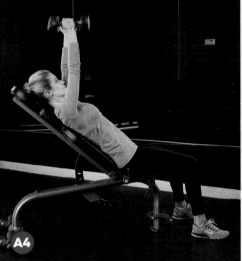

WALKING LUNGE
Step forward on one leg, bending both knees as you go down. Keep about 2 feet between each foot. Lower body and drive front knee over toe, touching hamstring to calf and keeping heel flat. Return to starting position on the same path used to lower, and alternate legs.

45-DEGREE DUMBBELL PRESS
Start with dumbbells in a neutral position. Push straight up without touching dumbbells at top. As you lower dumbbells, pinch shoulder blades together while having elbows track out at a 45-degree angle.

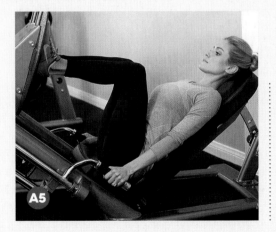

LEG PRESS
Start with feet just outside shoulder width, toes slightly pointed out. Cover weight as far as possible, letting knees track out slightly. To return to starting position, push evenly through both feet without allowing heels to come off platform.

Burning Calories Workout Chart

		DATE:		DATE:		DATE:		DATE:		DATE:	
		Weight	Time	Weight	Time	Weight	Time	Weight	Time	Weight	Time
A1 SQUATS WITH DUMBBELLS Time: 60 seconds	Set 1										
	Set 2										
	Set 3										
	Set 4										
	Set 5										
A2 SEATED ROW Time: 60 seconds	Set 1										
	Set 2										
	Set 3										
	Set 4										
	Set 5										
A3 WALKING LUNGE Time: 60 seconds	Set 1										
	Set 2										
	Set 3										
	Set 4										
	Set 5										
A4 45-DEGREE DUMBBELL PRESS Time: 60 seconds	Set 1										
	Set 2										
	Set 3										
	Set 4										
	Set 5										
A5 LEG PRESS Time: 60 seconds	Set 1										
	Set 2										
	Set 3										
	Set 4										
	Set 5										

The Nap Time Workout

For the first few months after I had Jaxon, the only working out I did was at home. I was able to squeeze in 30-minute sessions four or fives times a week, keeping the pace up to burn calories to get off that extra baby fat. Now if I'm alone with the kids, I'll still work out at home while the babies nap. Quick moves I love include:

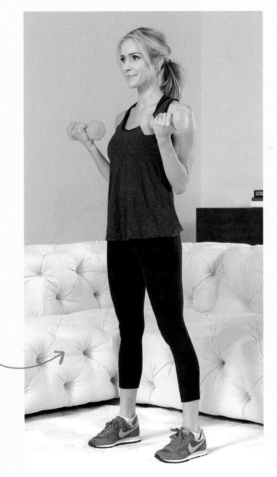

▶ **LUNGES:** 10 standing lunges each leg and 12 side lunges each leg.

▶ **SQUATS AGAINST THE WALL:** Hold for 30 seconds. Take a 60-second break, then repeat twice more.

▶ **LEG LIFTS WITH ANKLE WEIGHTS:** 30 lifts per leg.

▶ **BICYCLE ABS MOVE** (I do this in Pilates and love it): Lying on the floor and with your hands behind your neck, cross your elbow over to your opposite hip. Alternate sides, doing 30 altogether.

▶ **ARM-STRENGTHENING MOVES:** Shoulder press, biceps curl, lying-down triceps dips, and bent-over lateral raise. Do 18 reps each with whatever weight you are comfortable with (I usually use 10 to 12 pounds).

Balancing It All

Because working out is a priority of mine, I will always make the time. For example, before kids, I used to get a manicure and pedicure every week. But I can count the number of times I have done that since becoming a mom, because I just don't care enough about that anymore. Having my nails look good is no longer enough of a concern to make it worth the time. But working out, feeling good, and being healthy are my main priorities.

Making the time can be tough, though. There are days when it's just me and my kiddos and they are driving me up the wall, and working out is the last thing I want to do. But even getting the blood flowing for 30 minutes during nap time or with them playing next to me makes me feel better. Camden loves working out with me—he puts on ankle bands and kicks his legs. It's pretty darn cute. Traveling means I'm usually working out two or three times a week; a week home means four or five sessions that week. If I work out only 2 days a week, I don't stress about that low number like I used to. I simply keep eating clean and dedicate myself to going more frequently the following week. I take the weekends off because it's important to give your body a rest (and it's a nice mental break to know you can relax!).

Number of hours or days a week aside, exercising represents something I do for myself that makes me feel good in myriad ways. I'm proud of having a constant goal that is so positive. Through consistency and dedication, working out (along with eating well) has made me truly healthy.

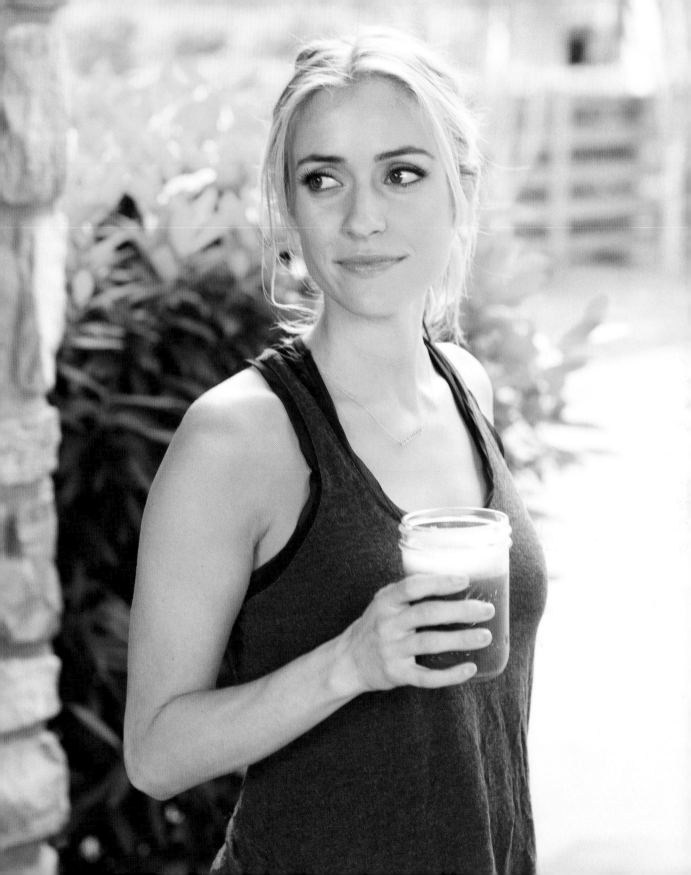

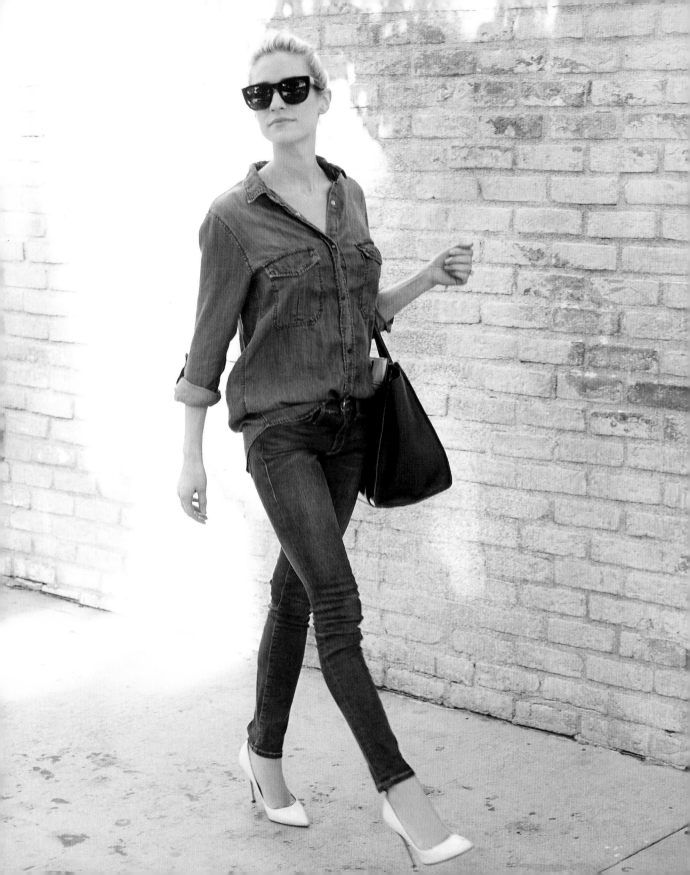

5

Find Your Fashion

MY FASHION PHILOSOPHY IS SIMPLE: THERE ARE NO RULES.
Fashion doesn't have to be intimidating or overwhelming. And it definitely doesn't have to cost a fortune. Fashion is fun and creative. It's an opportunity to convey something about yourself and feel good. What you wear is often the first thing people notice about you, so you want your clothes and accessories to be an expression of who you are.

I used to think fashion was only about the latest trends, and that to be stylish I had to conform to those particular styles. Makes sense, right? But it's not true. Learning from some great stylists, and through trial and error, I've realized the best looks are all about what looks best on my body. Working with my body type and flattering my features give me the confidence to pull off anything I like—and that self-assurance is often the key to looking great.

COME A LONG WAY

I wasn't always interested in fashion. In high school, high-end designers were never on my radar. I didn't really understand what fashion was. All I knew was that my Miss Sixty jeans were pretty damn cool. Between my platform sandals, black choker (*Laguna Beach* fans, you know what I'm talking about!), and jean skirts, I thought I looked pretty good!

Once I moved up to Los Angeles at age 18, I was thrust into a glamorous world of photo shoots and events, where I was dressed by stylists in the most beautiful clothes. I quickly became aware of who Alexander McQueen and Marc Jacobs were. Because of these different events and more jobs in TV, I was led to a few different stylists. The first stylist I worked with put me in what *she* wanted me to wear, not what *I* wanted to wear. She decked me out in mostly super-girly dresses. One time, I complained that a particular dress was made for an ice-skater: frilly with lots of movement and a huge cutout on the chest (nowadays I like more structure). But ultimately, I was too young and naive to say no, so I went along with her choices, unhappy the entire time. A different stylist wanted me to wear only trendy pieces, even though half of them didn't flatter my body. This resulted in a lot of uncomfortable moments because I didn't feel good in the clothes. I worked with a few other stylists, some who I loved, and some who were just okay. I saw all types of different perspectives and wore a *ton* of different clothes. Not only was I grateful for all of this exposure, but I learned a lot about myself and about fashion in general.

> What all these experiences taught me was what I like and what I don't like. I figured out my body type and what looks the best on me. Trendy doesn't always mean flattering!

Most of all, what all these experiences taught me was what I like and what I don't like. I figured out my body type and what looks the best on me. Trendy doesn't always mean flattering! I'm 5 foot 3 and petite, and I literally have no hips, so it's easy for me to get swallowed in clothes. Since I'm so short, I can't wear skirts

The Best Tips I've Picked Up from Stylists

▸ **TAILORING IS EVERYTHING.** It does take a little extra money, but it makes your clothes fit perfectly. Since I'm so small, most of my clothes need tailoring; otherwise they're too long or big in certain areas. An item that looks just okay can be transformed by a great tailor. Taking skirts in at the bottom to make them slightly tighter is one of the best tricks. It instantly makes them more flattering on everyone.

▸ **ALWAYS TRY CLOTHES ON.** Clothes look different on hangers. Stylists have insisted that I try on certain dresses and shorts that I've been sure wouldn't look good on me, and I've ended up loving them.

▸ **STEP OUT OF YOUR COMFORT ZONE.** It's good to explore different styles of clothes in case you stumble upon something you actually like! I've been persuaded to try clothes I never thought I would like in a million years, and sometimes I've been pleasantly surprised. For example, if you always wear skinny jeans, try on a pair of boyfriend jeans to change things up once in a while. With the right outfit, they could end up being your new favorites.

▸ **TAKE A PICTURE OF YOURSELF IN YOUR OUTFIT.** This is better than a mirror because it truly shows you what the ensemble looks like. You're able to be more objective about an outfit when you aren't looking in a mirror. Also, color changes a lot in photos, due to what your background is and what the lighting is like. For example, when I'm mixing and layering neutrals, like a certain cream with white, a picture will tell me whether the subtle color changes work or clash.

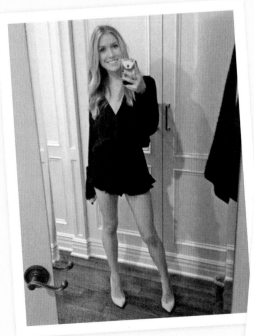

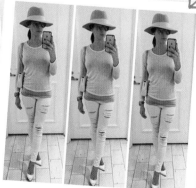

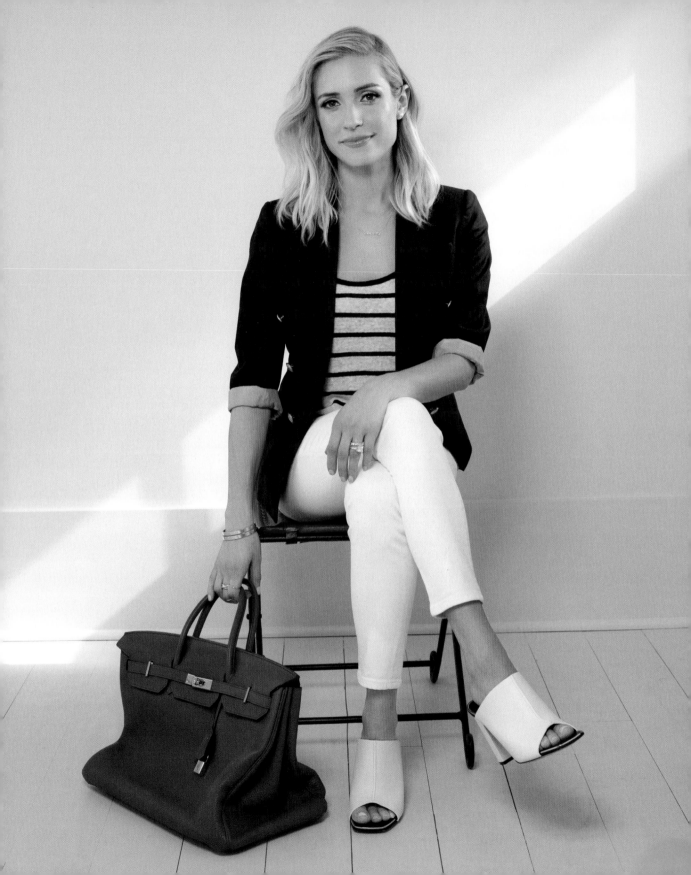

that fall below my knees unless they are full length. I also need clothes that are fitted and not too loose. I love shift dresses, but unless I get them tailored, they swallow me. I am drawn to things that give me some shape: rompers and jumpers because they have a waist, and skinny jeans. Now when I use stylists, I'm able to express my wants and tell them what to avoid. (Good stylists know these things right away when they first meet me, though.) When I was young, before I knew my body, I didn't have the first clue about what to wear (or say no to). Now I've figured out what I like and what looks good on me, so even when I'm working with someone else, I'm able to make fashion an expression of who I am instead of someone else's idea of me.

MY STYLE

My personal style is about structure and simplicity. I love looking effortless, like I just threw my outfit together in 2 minutes flat. I love flexible clothes, meaning the majority of my clothes look great with everything else in my closet. And nothing too girly. I stick mostly to neutrals, occasionally adding a pop of color with shoes or a bag. You will find mostly black, white, and gray in my closet. I know what I like, and I stick to it. I like to layer shirts, for example, to make a minimal look more dynamic. In general, I keep to great jeans, structured dresses, and basics. Then I add flare with accessories—understated jewelry, a great pair of shoes, and a nice bag. Nothing too over the top. I love hats, belts, and all shoes, of course. With the right pair of shoes, you can make any simple outfit chic. My favorite outfit is one with layered basics: a tank top and long-sleeved shirt, jeans, booties, a belt, a hat, and sunglasses. Easy, classy, and (seemingly) effortless. Those basic pieces can be worn a million different ways and over and over without hesitation, since they're neutral and for everyday wear.

My Favorite Outfits

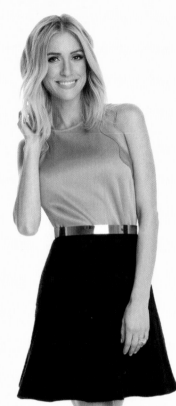

▶ Blue isn't a color I normally wear but I love how soft and sweet this is paired with the flirty skirt and pink heels.

▶ I love incorporating a pop of color with shoes when wearing a solid color.

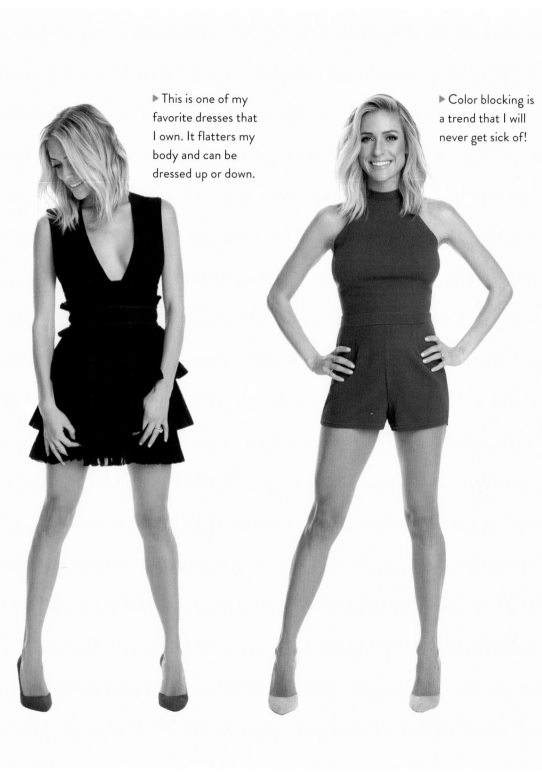

▶ This is one of my favorite dresses that I own. It flatters my body and can be dressed up or down.

▶ Color blocking is a trend that I will never get sick of!

WHAT TO WEAR AND HOW TO WEAR IT

Five Key Pieces, Three Different Ways

I'm all about making the most out of your closet and each piece individually. To maximize the pieces I already own, it's important to think outside of the box about how to wear each item. One point to consider is that two disparate things (whether it be two different types of fabric or two pieces that are tonally different, like a floral dress with a leather jacket) can sometimes create fashion harmony. Layering—sweaters with button-down shirts, and button-downs with blazers—also creates different looks from the same core pieces. Accessories, especially shoes, go a long way in changing the mood of an outfit—see Accessories That Make the Look (page 155) for some ideas. Below are some of my favorite items that I wear time and time again and how I use them to create different looks.

1 **BLACK LEATHER PANTS.** There's nothing I love more than leather pants! They're an obvious choice for a night out, but they look chic during the day too. I actually think they're sexier when dressed down. I've worn mine with heels and a big, chunky sweater to lunch. They look great with booties, a white tank, and a blazer. For a dressier look, any kind of top—a sheer blouse, a backless top, a sexy sleeveless shirt— looks good with leather pants and simple, pointy-toe heels. Make sure the fit is snug, since leather pants tend to stretch slightly.

2 **BOOTIES.** My favorite kind of shoe! I love them because they are so versatile. Wear them with dresses (short, or long and casual, or dressy), jeans for running around, and flirty skirts for a dinner out. Booties make any outfit chic.

3 **WHITE BLAZER.** I love blazers. A white one looks clean and fresh. Wear it with a pretty, feminine dress or romper to lunch with the girls. I've worn my white blazer with jeans (I've even worn it with another key piece, leather pants) or jean shorts for running errands.

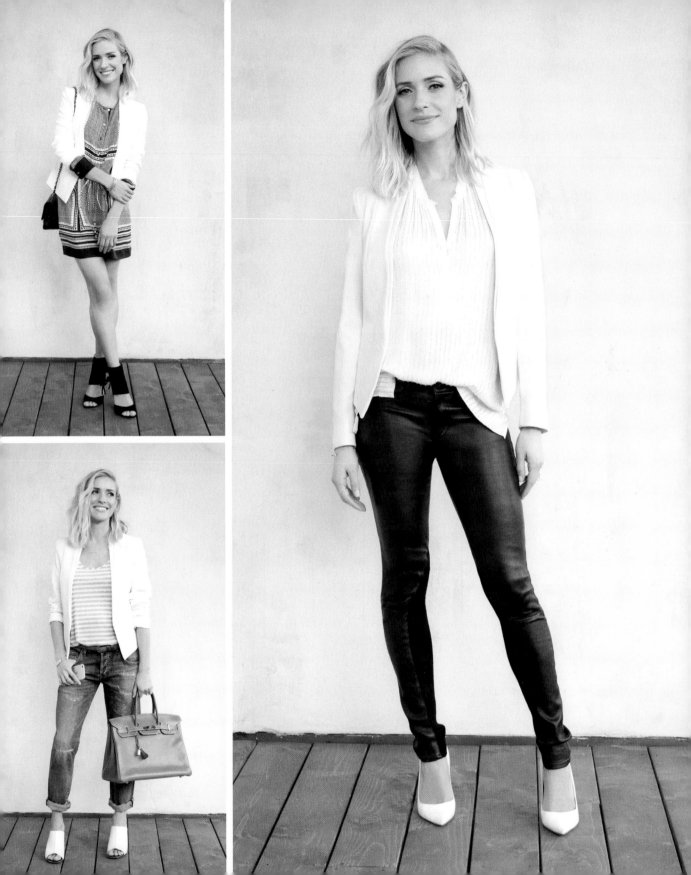

4 **JUMPERS.** These might be my favorite pieces because they're so easy: Not a lot of thought needs to go into wearing them besides selecting accessories. I love wearing a jumper with a wedge heel to brunch or with flats for running around with the kids. For a night out, heels and a blazer look classy.

5 **ARMY GREEN JEAN SHORTS.** I like army green shorts because they're slightly different (I also love white)—they feel more fun than the everyday blue jean shorts. I love the look of jean shorts with flats, a T-shirt, belt, and hat for the daytime. A sandal heel and blouse go nicely with jean shorts for a casual dinner. If you are at the beach, just pair them with your bathing suit top and sunglasses.

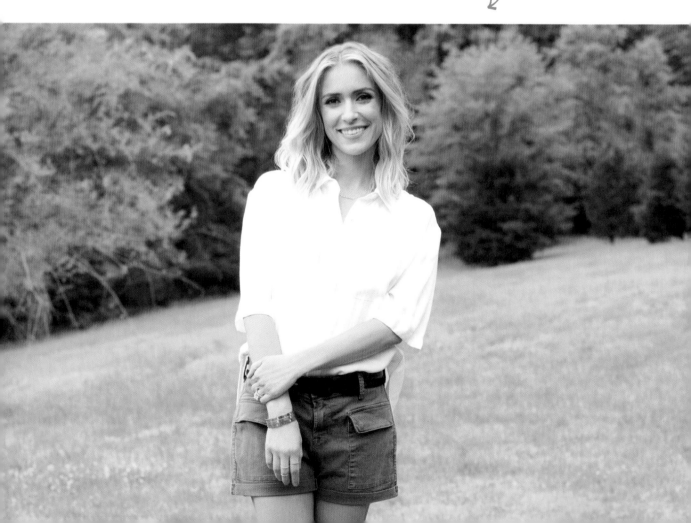

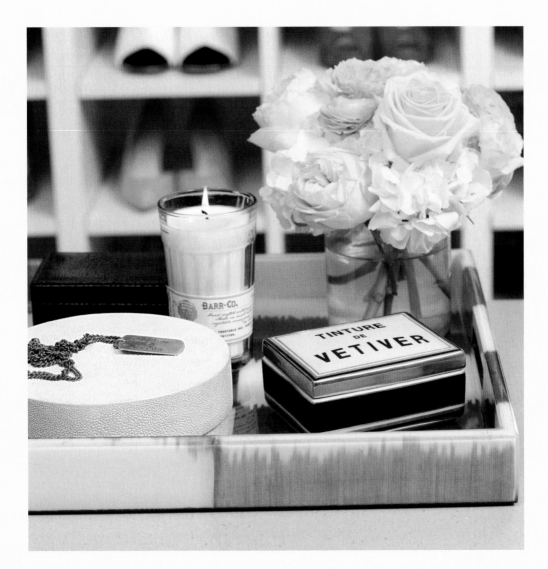

Simplicity doesn't apply only to my fashion sense regarding clothes. It also drives the way I decorate my home. I don't like anything too cluttered or busy, and I don't want anything to ever look too "done" or overthought. I keep everything—from decor to pieces of furniture—clean, simple, and mostly neutral. I would describe my home style as traditional with some rustic touches. I add feminine flair with candles and flowers.

My Top Essentials That Every Woman Should Own

There are a few key pieces that I think every woman needs in her closet. These staples will be with you for the rest of your life, since they're timeless and can be worn multiple ways.

1 **NUDE HEELS.** They elongate your legs when worn with any dress or skirt. They also go well with jeans and almost any color pant.

2 **LEATHER HANDBAG.** You only need one good one, so go for a neutral-colored bag that can be worn with everything. Leather is easier to clean and looks great with any outfit. I would get a medium-size bag to fit all your essentials like makeup when you're in your carefree twenties, and then to hold diapers and wipes when you have kids. Plus, that size is perfect for traveling because you can slip in a book and a scarf, even a snack!

3 **WHITE PETER PAN COLLAR SLEEVELESS SHIRT.** This can be worn by itself with jeans and heels, tucked into a skirt, or under a sweater with the collar sticking out. It also goes well with a blazer and jeans. This piece will never go out of style.

4 **SKINNY BLACK BELT WITH A GOLD BUCKLE.** I have one that I've punched extra holes in so I can wear it around my waist or hips. I wear mine with everything from dresses and skirts to jeans. Everyone needs one good, versatile belt. I like the touch of gold since it makes it slightly dressier than just a plain black belt. If you wear silver more often, then go for that.

5 **BLACK ANKLE-STRAP HEELS.** A black heel is a must for every girl, as you can wear it with anything from dresses to jeans. I like one with an ankle strap since it gives it a little extra spice. Ankle straps are sexy and bring an edgy touch to any outfit.

6 **BROWN FLOPPY-BRIM HAT.** I have a Rag and Bone one that I live in. I've worn mine on the beach and to lunch with girlfriends. Hats bring ultimate style to any outfit without trying too hard.

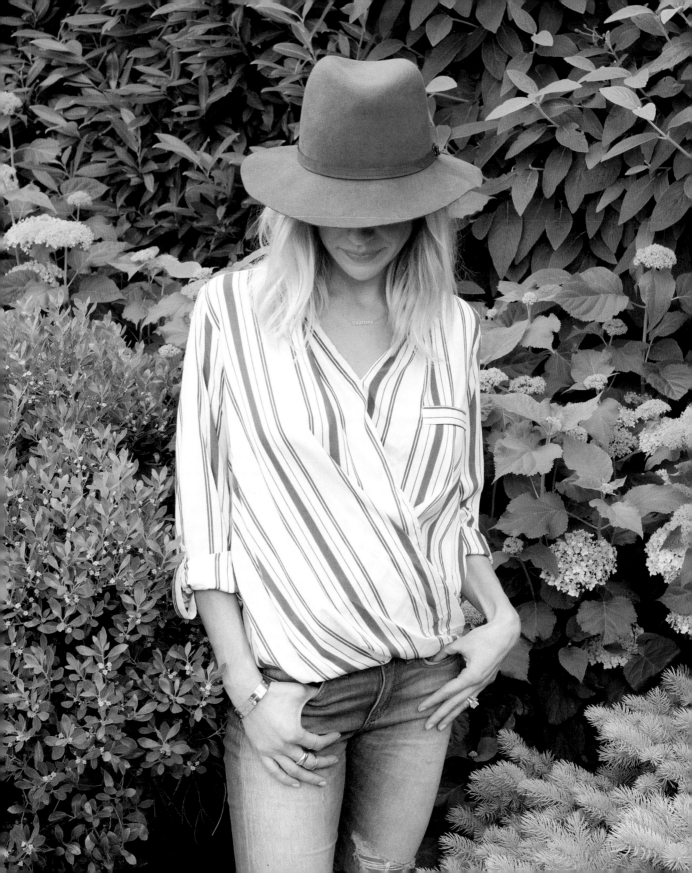

When to Splurge

A few items are worth spending some money on. Certain things cannot be shortchanged—you can tell when they aren't the real deal. When it's a garment you will have in your closet forever, it's worth the expense.

▶ **BLACK LEATHER JACKET.** You'll need to keep a few things in mind when shopping for this item. Go for a classic black, since colored leather goes in and out of style. Black is timeless and can be worn multiple ways. Search for a jacket that will improve with age—you want one that looks good worn in. I have one that looks better every year as it becomes more distressed. Stay away from embellishments, since these are easy to get sick of and your taste may change down the road.

▶ **LBD (LITTLE BLACK DRESS).** The perfect LBD is neither too long nor too short, so it's superflexible. Just above the knees makes it appropriate for most occasions and is easily dressed up or down. You want one that is simple enough that you can change up the look with different accessories and jackets. Look for a fabric that can be worn year-round (sorry, velvet) and that looks good worn with or without tights. Don't go for trends (cutouts, ruffles, etc.) because those change rapidly. Classy never fades.

▶ **THE PERFECT PAIR OF JEANS.** You need only one pair of amazing jeans. They need to fit you perfectly, so be willing to try on a million pairs and jump on the ones that make you feel great.

The perfect pair looks good dressed up or down and flatters your body. Don't get a pair that's too trendy with patterns. Instead, go for a dark denim since it can be dressed up. For me, the perfect pair are skinnies, not too tight or too loose: They need to be appropriate for dinner with the in-laws, a business meeting, and kicking around doing errands. Mine are often too long when I purchase them, and they need to be tailored. If jeans need shortening, don't let this stop you from buying them! If their length is the only thing making you hesitate, pay a little extra to have them taken up. It's worth it!

▶ **ONE GOOD SET OF LINGERIE.** Only if this is your thing! I like lingerie because it makes me feel sexy and gives me something to get excited about. I would be lying if I said I wear it all the time. I used to have this vision of myself always looking cute in lingerie and little nighties. That's just not the case! I love my sweatpants and leggings too much. But when I do wear lingerie, it feels special. One great set that I will love forever is plenty for me, but if you are a big lingerie girl, then go ahead and get as many as you want! Whatever makes you happy!

Save That Money, Honey

There are a lot of pieces in my closet that I hardly ever spend real money on. I'm a huge fan of buying trendier pieces at more inexpensive places since they'll only be worn for a season or two.

▸ **DIAMOND EARRINGS.** It's rare that I wear earrings, except when I dress up, and then sometimes I wear fake diamonds (especially when I travel). Some people think I'm silly for this, but I'm all for it! I lost a real diamond earring in high school, and I'm still heartbroken over it. Wearing fakes means I won't get as upset if I accidentally lose one. No one can tell the difference anyway!

▸ **BLAZERS.** My favorite black blazer is from Topshop (where it certainly cost under $100, if I remember correctly), and you would never know the difference between it and a super-expensive designer blazer. I love saving on blazers, because then you can buy some in trendier colors and styles. I have a bright yellow blazer that I've only worn a handful of times, but I don't mind since it wasn't expensive.

▸ **BELTS.** I would put money on the fact that no one will ever be able to guess where your belt came from. The style of belts comes and goes, so buy inexpensive ones and have fun with the different designs.

▸ **BASIC SHIRTS.** Every single basic shirt you own—tanks, tees, long sleeved—should be inexpensive. Mine get stains on them from the kids, so I can't justify paying a lot. Also, plain, simple, inexpensive shirts are often imperceptibly different than designer ones.

A simple yet chic outfit with basics

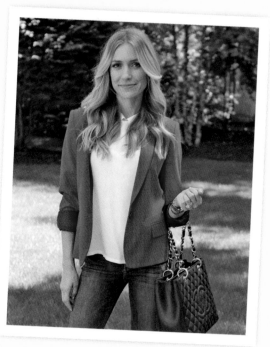

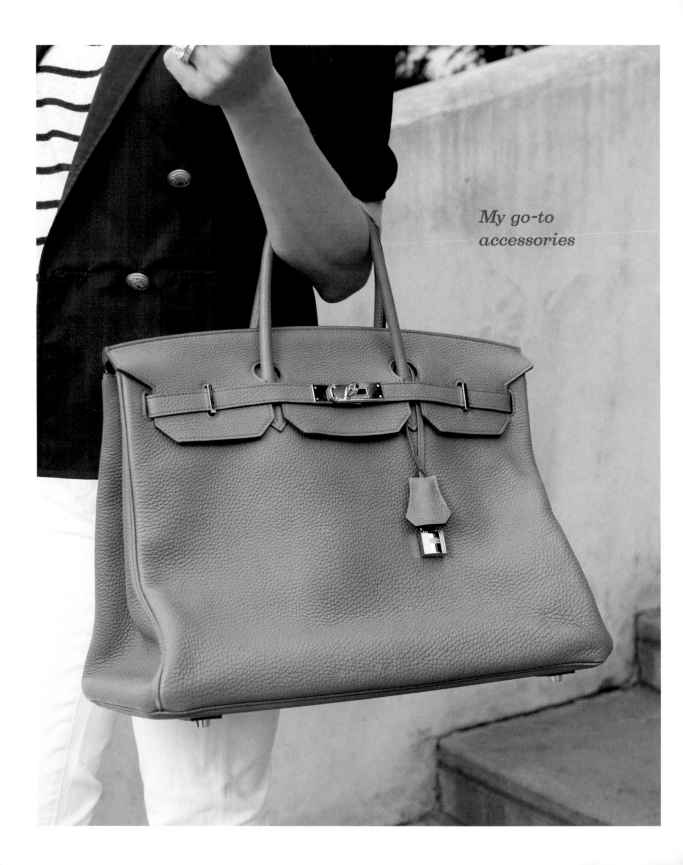

My go-to accessories

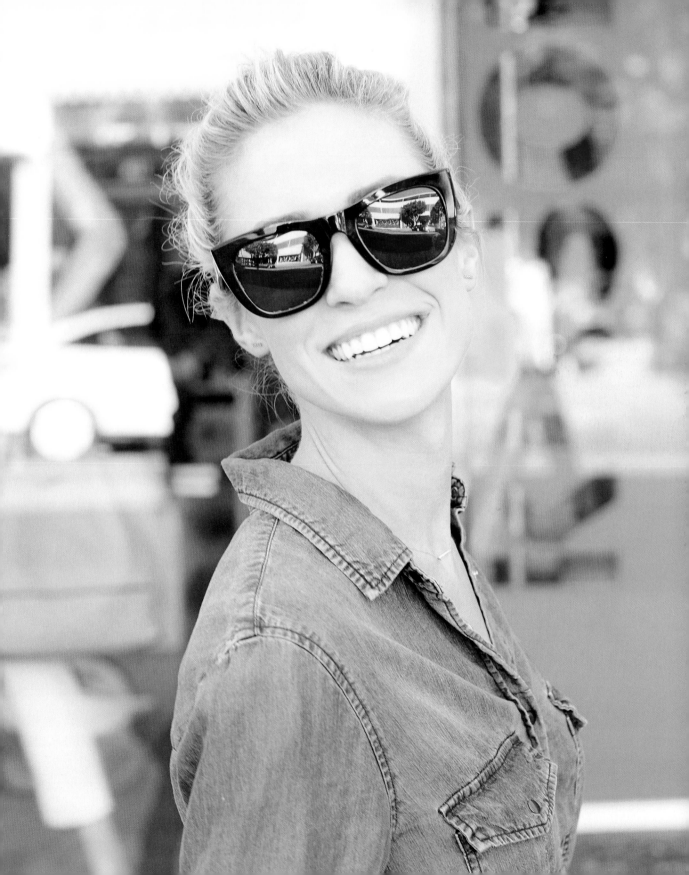

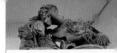
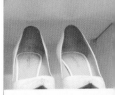
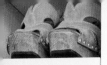
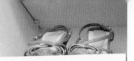
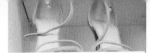
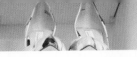
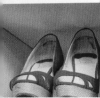
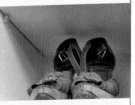
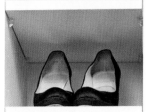
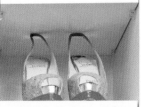
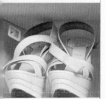
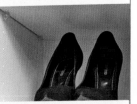
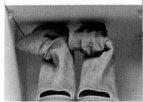
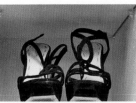
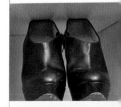
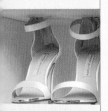
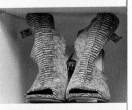
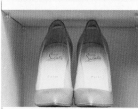
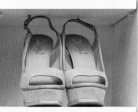
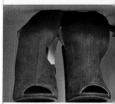
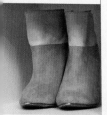
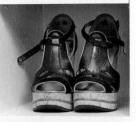
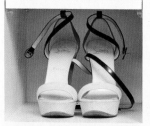
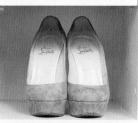
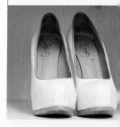
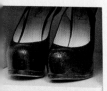
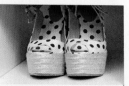
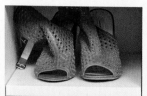
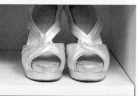
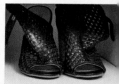
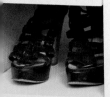
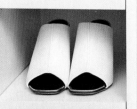
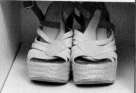
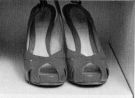
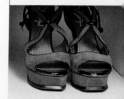
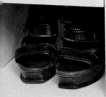
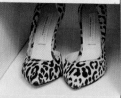
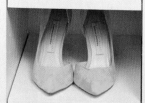
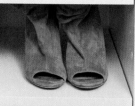
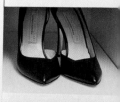
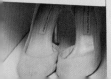
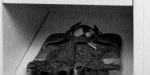
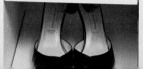
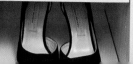
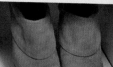

Accessories That Make the Look

Like I've said before, accessories can make an otherwise basic outfit look great. Belts, hats, and sunglasses are more often a part of my outfits than not. Focusing on accessories to take an outfit to the next level keeps getting dressed fairly easy and painless.

▶ **JEWELRY** brings an extra element to every outfit. With a big statement necklace, you can let the jewelry do the talking—it can be enough with an otherwise simple dress or tee and skinny jeans. For everyday, I wear a few small rings and two or three layered necklaces (dainty ones, of course) or sometimes just a watch with one simple bangle. As I noted earlier, it's rare that I wear earrings, for no particular reason. I also don't wear earrings, necklace, rings, and bracelets at the same time. I never want to look too done. I usually pick two, maybe three, pieces to wear, but never all four. If I wear a statement necklace, I keep everything else clean or only wear simple studs and/or rings.

▶ **SHOES** make or break an outfit. They also have the ability to instill confidence instantly, giving you extra height and longer legs (maybe that's the 5-foot-3-inch part of me talking!). With the right shoes, I feel sexy and like I can take on anything. Plus, they change the mood of an outfit immediately. Slipping on heels instantly dresses up an outfit, and changing from a solid-color, closed-toe heel to a sexy, strappy sandal or bold print heel transitions the same outfit from work to play in a second. I love putting an outfit together around my shoes. Working from the bottom up gives direction to the outfit and keeps outfits looking fresh, since different shoes completely change the look and feel of an outfit you have already worn. In that way, shoes help maximize the clothes you have in your closet.

True confession: There are very few shoes I don't like! I love everything from classic nude pumps to slouchy boots to pointy flats. Suede is by far my favorite fabric for shoes. I think colors look so rich and luxurious when done in beautiful suede. Leather is classic and can be worn with anything. I like prints (such as a floral) in leather for a glossy finish. Shoes are my icing on the cake—the best part!

BEING THE OPPOSITE OF A HOARDER

I'm slightly obsessed with getting rid of stuff. There's nothing I like doing more than going through the refrigerator and getting rid of old condiments and food. The same goes for my closet. I go through my wardrobe about once a month and bag clothes that I know I'm not going to wear. (I always let my friends have first dibs before I donate them.) Going through a closet once a month may seem insane—I know, I know. But I'm in fashion. I go shopping a lot and get sent clothes all the time! It's one of the perks, and I'm truly lucky for that. If you're not as type A as I am, set a goal to go through your closet at least twice a year, ideally in the beginning of spring and fall. The idea is to weed out everything that you don't like, that doesn't fit, or that is worn out. While you are at it, put away any off-season clothes and bring out seasonally appropriate things from last year. Every spring, I store my big sweaters in airtight bags that shrink down to almost nothing, and

Taking Care of Clothes

▸ Wash your jeans as little as necessary. Hang and air them between wearings—don't toss them in a pile or smash them into a drawer. I honestly have no clue exactly how many times I wash my jeans a year, but I would guess I could count it on both hands. The only time I wash them is when they smell or have dirt or stains on them. Doing this makes them last longer.

▸ Invest in a small steamer. I bought a little one that I bring when I travel. I like steamers better than irons because they don't leave any creases and are super-easy and fast to use.

▸ Make sure to read garment labels and get important sweaters and shirts dry-cleaned. I'm still not over a sweater that I shrank years ago. It was an open cardigan in the perfect beige that went with everything. The first time I washed it, it shrank to fit a doll! So take care how you choose to clean your favorite things, since washing at home could cause some damage.

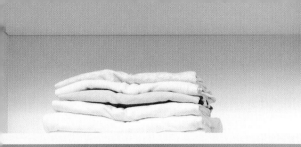
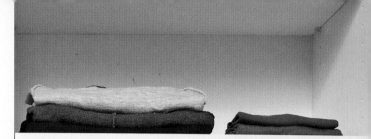
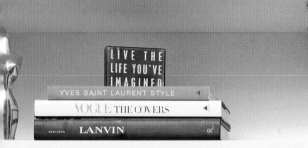

LIVE THE
LIFE YOU'VE
IMAGINED

YVES SAINT LAURENT STYLE

VOGUE THE COVERS

MERCERON LANVIN

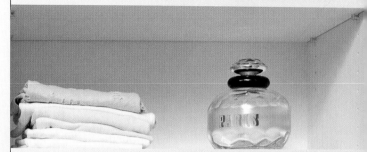
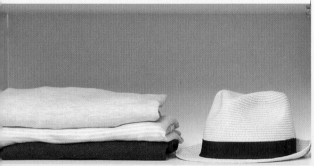
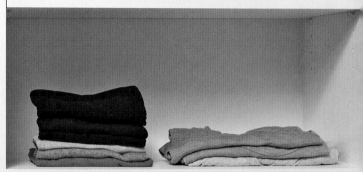
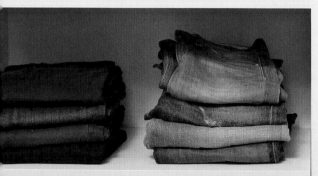
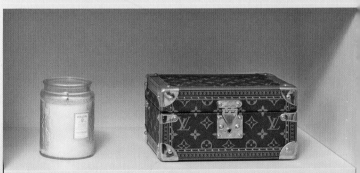
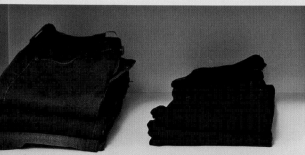
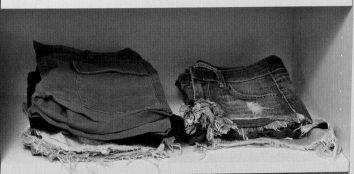

stack them in a guest room closet. Then, come fall, since I haven't seen those clothes in months, they feel new again. Well, almost!

Sometimes I struggle with getting rid of a certain piece that I really love but haven't worn in a year. If I'm on the fence, I'll allow myself to hold on to it, but if I still haven't worn it by the next time I clean out my closet, then it's time to part ways!

A frequently cleaned closet makes getting dressed simple and easy. It keeps everything organized and creates more room for new garments you love. Plus, it declutters your shelves so you can see everything you own. Having stuff that you don't wear in your field of vision can be super-distracting. When you have fewer things to choose from, putting an outfit together is that much easier.

THINGS YOU SHOULD DEFINITELY GET RID OF

▶ Anything that you haven't worn in more than 2 years. If you haven't worn it by now, you never will, and it's distracting to keep it in your closet. Give it to a friend who will love it and get great use out of it.

▶ Any T-shirts or sweaters you have from ex-boyfriends. Why are you still holding on to those? Time to move on and ditch 'em.

▶ Things that you like/love but can't figure out for the life of you how to wear. I bought a beautiful baby-pink leather jacket, but I've had a hard time putting it together with anything, even though it looked great in the store. (Full disclosure: I haven't gotten the courage to get rid of this yet. I'm giving myself one more season to find the perfect outfit for it!)

▶ Any color that isn't flattering on you. Olive green tops are horrible on me. (I can get away with shorts, but shirts look terrible.) We all have at least one bad color, so be honest with yourself and move on.

▶ Bridesmaid dresses that you haven't worn since the wedding. I've been able to wear only one again. Like everything else in your closet, if it's been over 2 years and the garment hasn't seen daylight, it's time to say goodbye.

▶ Old underwear. When they have little holes and stains (oh, come on, we all get them), it's time to throw them out!

Packing for Trips

Since I live on planes, I'm constantly packing a suitcase. I like taking as little as possible, ideally not even checking a bag. Different kinds of trips require different essentials. Here is what I make sure to pack.

▶ **BEACH VACAY:** Two bikinis: one string and one bandeau to even out the tan lines. A great pair of flats that can be dressed up or down, a neutral heel, and a floppy-brim hat. Lots of basics: tanks, shorts, long-sleeved shirts for when it gets chilly, and a couple of simple dresses. I like bringing dainty jewelry (a small necklace or a couple of simple rings) for the beach and one big statement necklace to wear with a plain dress.

▶ **NEW YORK CITY BUSINESS TRIP:** Solid-color blazer (usually black) and a fun, flirty skirt to wear with the blazer to meetings. At night, I remove the blazer and switch my booties to heels for dinner with girlfriends. New York is the place for a bold necklace, so I bring an outfit that works well with one.

▶ **L.A. BUSINESS TRIP:** Basics: tanks to layer with T-shirts or simple long sleeved shirts and skinny jeans. A romper or jumper to wear with a light jean jacket or blazer. Booties, hats, sunglasses. I usually bring one pair of workout shoes and leggings, a sports bra, and a tank top. If I have time, I work out when I travel, even if it means I can only squeeze in 30 minutes (see Chapter 4).

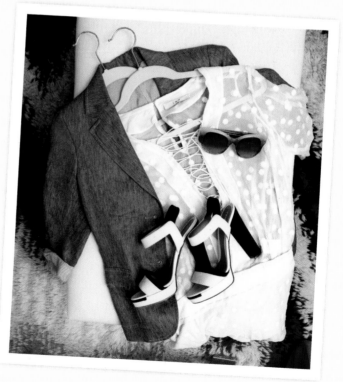

Balancing It All

In short, for me, fashion is about being myself. Knowing my body and what looks good on it makes all the difference. With that knowledge, shopping is much easier—I don't struggle to figure out my style and question if I should wear a certain design or not. Now I know exactly what I like and what will look good. For fun, I occasionally try on clothes or accessories that I wouldn't normally wear on the off chance I might discover something that I never realized would look flattering.

Organization definitely helps me put outfits together. Keeping only my favorite and essential clothes makes getting dressed quick and painless. I have more time to be with my babies instead of picking through a pile of unworn garments. No one has time to try on 50 different outfits every morning. In my closet, I have a uniform of basics, a few special things, and booties, hats, and accessories to make anything look chic.

Confidence is a huge part of fashion. Feeling good in your skin goes a long way to feeling good in your clothes. Remember, clothes are often a way to say something about yourself, so let go of the shoulds and shouldn'ts and instead focus on feeling comfortable and confident.

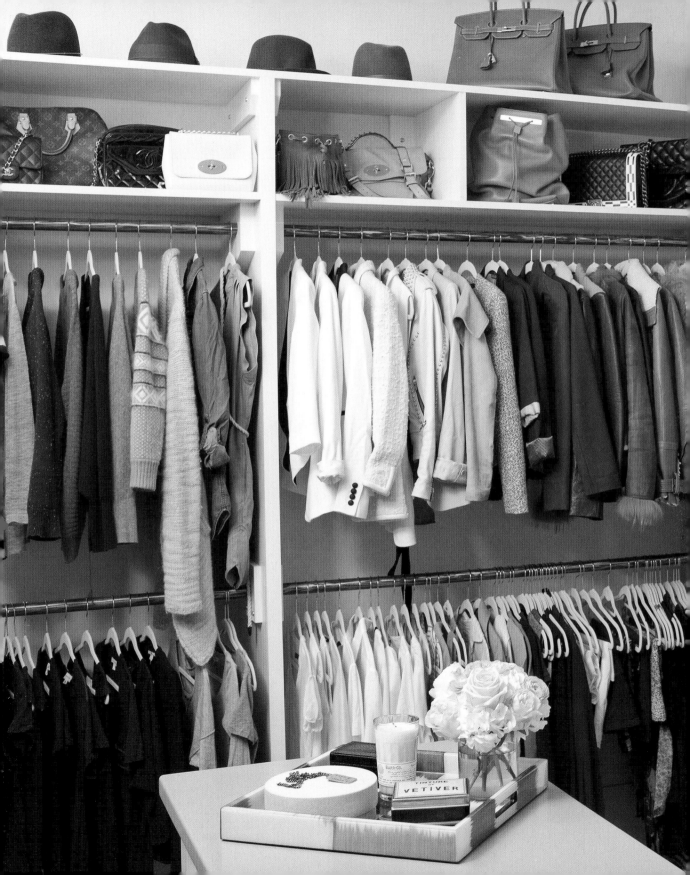

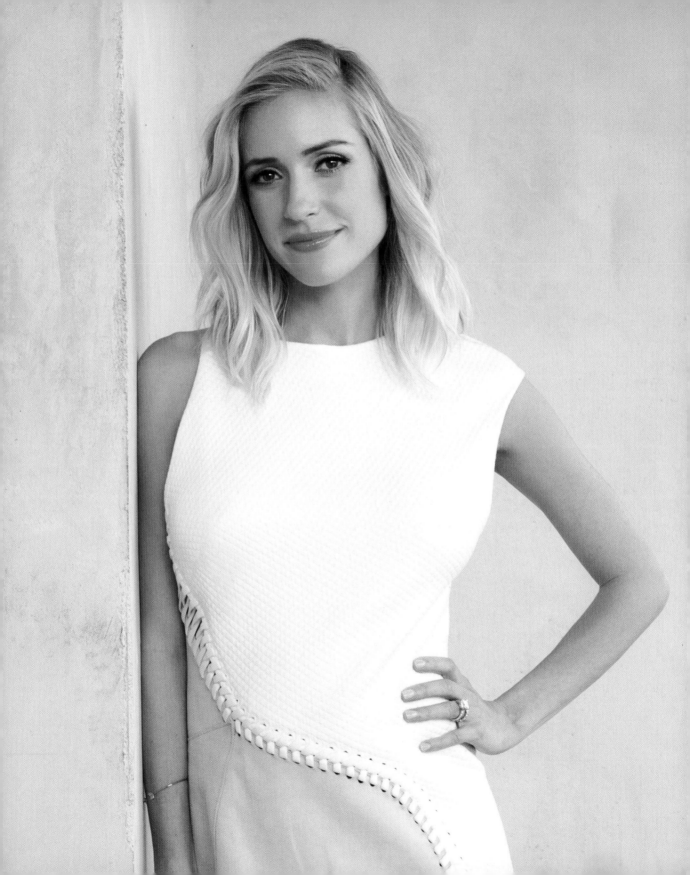

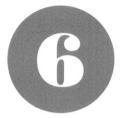

Glowing Girl

MY BEAUTY PHILOSOPHY CERTAINLY HAS EVOLVED SINCE MY teenage years. I look back to some high school pictures and say, "Ugh, what the heck was I thinking?!" I used to wear black eyeliner on the inside of my lower lids for a dramatic look every single day and felt naked without it. During my early high school years, my eyebrows were a mess from overplucking (I even plucked on top of the brow, which I now know is a no-no). I always had zits and wore fake nails. Always. Once, for a school dance, I got my makeup done and looked horrible. I had a pound of foundation and the biggest fake lashes they could find glued on my face. Not cute.

Over the years, the amount of cosmetics I wear daily has gradually diminished. These days, I keep my beauty routine simple and more natural. I'm just too lazy to do a full face of makeup every morning. Honestly, I find that caring about my appearance to that extent is exhausting, and that's 20 minutes I could be spending on something more productive. Maybe since I'm married and Jay likes me better without makeup, I unconsciously stopped caring as much. Having kids also doesn't give you the time to spend in front of a mirror! Plus, I've come to realize that less makeup is better for my skin.

So today, the most important part of my beauty routine is maintaining a healthy base, which for me is all about clear skin and maintained brows. Then for special events, when I want to supplement my look a little, I have a clean, healthy face to work with.

My hair, on the other hand, is a bit of an obsession. While I don't necessarily spend a great deal of time on it, I do feel much better when I've got a good blowout than when my locks are tied back in a ponytail. It's my vice, what can I say.

THE MANE

My hair is my most important cosmetic adornment. With great hair, I'm on top of the world. When I was really little, a psychic told my mom that I would be obsessed with my hair. Boy, was she right!

::

ON PSYCHICS

I'm just like my mom when it comes to psychics. We love them, we don't take them too seriously, but sometimes they are spot-on with certain things! The psychic reading is more entertainment than anything. That said, the psychic who my mom consulted when I was a child clearly saw right through me. She also told my mom that my passport would get great use. Right and right!

Maintenance

Since my hair takes a beating from constantly being styled for shoots and events, it's important to hydrate it often and give it a break when I'm not working. I try not to wash too often, which usually translates to only every 3 days. In between shampoos, I use dry shampoo. My hair actually styles better when it's not freshly washed. If I've washed it and need to make it look good, I use dry shampoo as a styling aid.

About once a month, I apply a hydrating mask made with coconut oil all over my scalp and on my hair from roots to ends. I leave it on for 30 minutes, then wash it out. Unlike olive oil or other heavy hair masks, coconut oil completely washes out with just one wash. (When I was in junior high, I put olive oil on my entire head, and it took almost a week to come out. I looked like a little grease ball!)

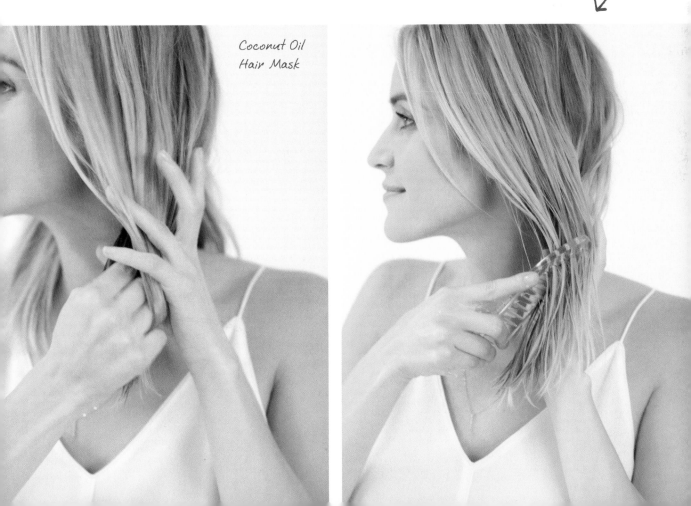

Coconut Oil
Hair Mask

I get my color done typically every 8 weeks. My hair is cut or trimmed every other coloring visit, meaning the haircut or trim is done usually every 3 to 4 months. I get highlights every other time and touch up my roots during the other visits. I don't mind when my hair looks a little "rooty," as my hair colorist calls it. As with everything else, I don't want my hair to look too perfect.

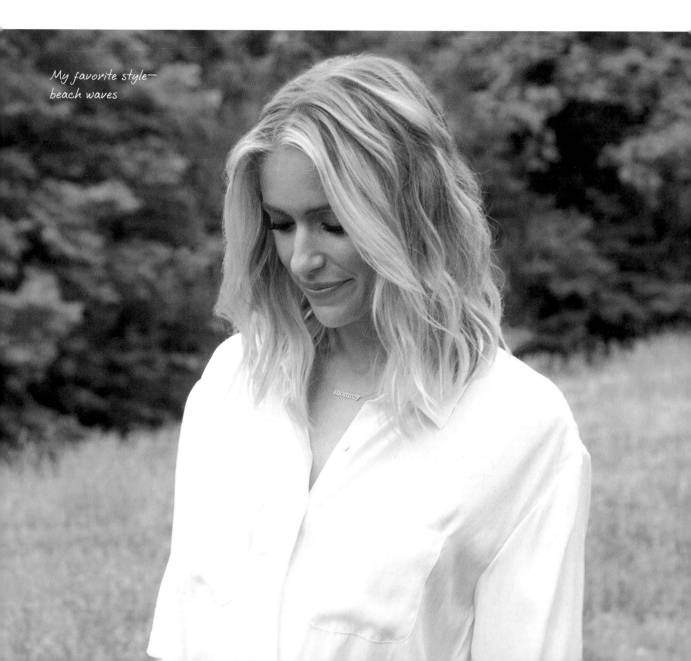

My favorite style—
beach waves

Styling

I'm predictable when it comes to my hair. I like it styled only a few ways, with my favorite being soft waves. Since I've cut my hair shorter, a side part has become my favorite look whether straight or waved. When my hair was long, I could go days without styling it and it still looked great. Now I have to take the time to style my hair if I want it to look decent. Short hair is definitely more work, but I like the change since my hair was long for so many years.

Perfecting beach waves can be tricky. It took me about 4 years before I was able to curl both sides of my head. For years, I could only make my left side look good!

Hair Tips from Scotty

Scotty Cuhna has been styling my hair for more than 5 years, and I've never worked with anyone better. He nails the sexy, undone look, and beach waves are his specialty. His top tips for styling your hair:

▶ Blondes should use a purple shampoo and conditioner because it takes out the brassiness without drying hair. You brunettes should use a shine or gloss treatment once a month if your hair gets a bit dull—your color will look more vibrant and healthy.

▶ To make waves or curls last another day, put your hair in a loose topknot with a scrunchie and wear it while you sleep. The next morning, add dry shampoo and shake out, don't brush. If you like, curl small sections with a small-barrel curling iron to freshen up the waves.

▶ To refresh bangs without ruining a blowout, spray bangs with a facial spray like Evian to restyle.

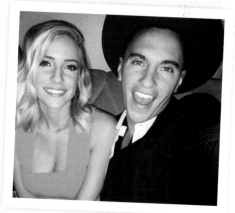

I prefer to start with unwashed hair, which holds the curl better. If I have to wash my hair but will be styling it with waves, I add dry shampoo. To get beachy waves, I put medium-size sections of hair flat between the two clamps of a flat iron, rotating and moving continuously. I shake them out when I've curled my whole head and spray with a texturizing spray. Sometimes I curl my hair going different directions to make the waves look more natural.

Volume isn't something that naturally happens for me, but I like volume no matter what style I'm doing: straight, beach waves, side part, or middle part. I have to work hard to get volume and make it last. This is why unwashed hair is truly better. I spray the roots with dry shampoo (that will instantly give it some volume) and tease underneath the top of my hair slightly. Texturizing spray helps keep hair thick throughout and gives it some shape.

SKIN

Good skin is where beauty starts. Growing up, I never had full-fledged acne, but I definitely had zits. It wasn't until I changed the way I ate that my skin completely transformed. Before, it was a miracle if I didn't have a zit, and now it's strange when I do. Obviously, a large part of that was due to hormones in my teenage years, but I had blemishes in my early twenties as well.

My goal is to never get Botox. Or any other filler or injectable, for that matter. I don't hate on people who get Botox; I would just prefer to do everything a more natural way. We don't know the long-term effects of that stuff, and it doesn't seem right to me. We are supposed to age—that's part of life! But for me, it's all about

::

HOMEMADE MOISTURIZING FACE MASK

This particular mask is great for the middle of winter when skin is dry and dull. I always have these two ingredients in the house, making the mask a piece of cake to whip up anytime.

Mash half an avocado and mix in 1 teaspoon honey. Apply to your face. Leave on for 10 minutes, then rinse off.

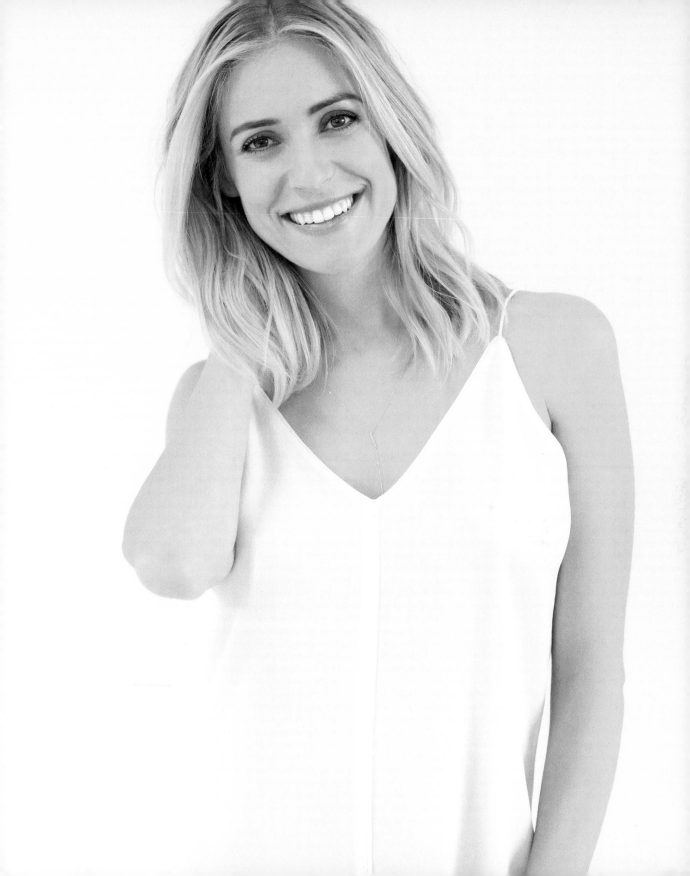

Homemade Coffee Face Scrub

Mix ¼ cup finely ground coffee beans and 2 tablespoons cocoa powder with either almond milk or melted coconut oil (start with 3 tablespoons and keep adding until you reach the desired consistency). Gently rub over your face (avoiding your eyes, of course), then rinse off; I use leftovers on my back and arms as well. Just make sure the coffee beans are finely ground to avoid scratching your face.

preventive care so that I can age naturally and gracefully. There are a lot of natural things you can do—and feel good about using—to help your skin look great.

It starts with what we put in our bodies. Once I started eating real food (see Chapter 3), my skin began to clear up and look fresh. In addition to following a healthy diet, I try to drink at least 90 ounces of water throughout the day. In fact, you won't see me without a water bottle! I believe this has a huge effect on keeping my face clear and hydrated.

Topically, my beauty routine is also all about hydration, hydration, hydration. Not long after I moved to Chicago and was breastfeeding my first son, Camden, I got a facial because I began breaking out again. The aesthetician told me that my skin was dehydrated. Even though I was drinking a ton of water, between the new cold weather and breastfeeding, it wasn't enough. She gave me a hydrating mask, which in my teens and early twenties I would have run from. So I started using the mask; sure enough, my skin improved. I use a mask to this day during winter months, and I notice a big difference. Just because I'm prone to breakouts doesn't mean I don't need some hydration love as well. A homemade mask (see "Homemade Moisturizing Face Mask," on page 168) is great because the ingredients are real, wholesome, and easy to find around the house. Just a few minutes wearing this mask can do wonders for your skin.

It's also important to do an exfoliating face scrub about once a week (see "Homemade Coffee Face Scrub," above). This removes dead skin cells, unclogs pores, and allows the skin to breathe.

I love rose hip oil for fighting fine lines and dryness. I squeeze a full dropper into my hands and rub all over my face at night. Another great product is coconut oil. I use this stuff for everything: cooking, baking, as a hair mask, and on my entire body. Some people swear by putting coconut oil on their entire face, but loading my face up with thick oil scares me a little (clearly those pimples as a teenager have scarred me a bit!). So I only apply it under my eyes and on my neck to help protect against aging and to hydrate.

Another product I swear by is vitamin C serum. I put it on a few nights a week to even out skin tone and combat any redness. It's also antiaging, because vitamin C is crucial for the production of collagen, helping maintain skin elasticity and firmness.

Preventive care for your skin also means using sunscreen. Take it from a girl who lived for many years in Southern California! I always use an SPF 30 organic sunscreen on my face. Some brands of sunscreen can be loaded with nasty chemicals, so it's important to look for a product with zinc oxide as the main ingredient. Fortunately, there are good options nowadays; you just have to read the ingredient labels like with everything else you buy.

Taking care of my skin means no matter how tired I am, I always remove my makeup and wash my face at night. There's nothing worse than waking up after sleeping in your makeup. My skin gets clogged after even one night. It's worth the 2 minutes!

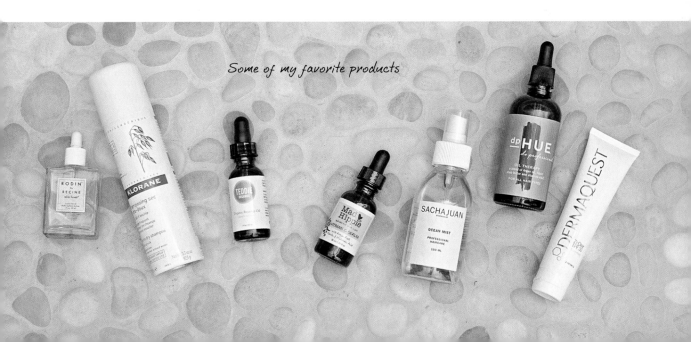

Some of my favorite products

BROWS

Brows frame the face and make a huge difference in appearance. I wasn't blessed with great brows, so I'm slightly obsessed with achieving really good ones. It's one of the first things I notice on other women, and I often have such brow envy!

I fill mine in slightly to create a full look. Since I'm blonde, I use a pencil that is slightly lighter than the color of my brows—I don't like them to look too dark, as that can be overpowering. It's best when brows are noticeable enough only to frame your face nicely. In junior high, I had the bright idea of plucking mine, but I had no clue what I was doing: I took a lot off the top (ahhh, such a bad move!) and made those babies teeny tiny. Needless to say, they looked awful. My mom's heart skipped a few beats when she first saw my hacked brows. When I was in high

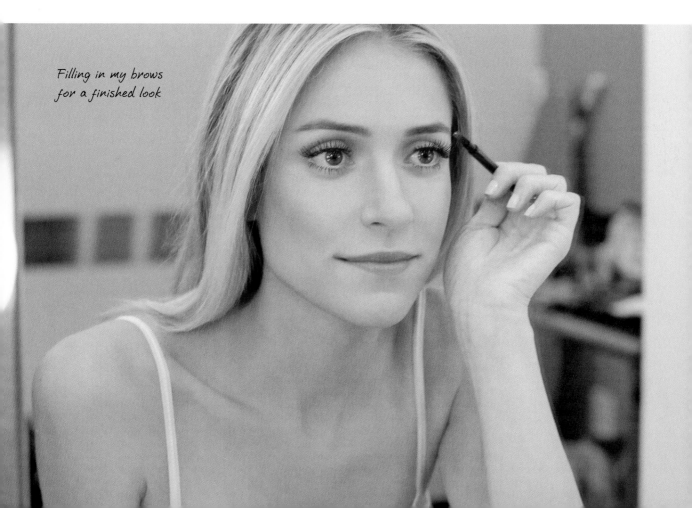

Filling in my brows
for a finished look

school, I had them groomed professionally and learned quite a bit in the process. The lady taught me never to pluck from the top, and she shaped them so that I could maintain them at home, getting them done professionally only a couple of times a year. Once I graduated from high school, I saw a girl regularly almost every month until I moved to Chicago. I fell prey to the L.A. idea that you need to get your brows done all the time, so I automatically did it when I got a bikini wax every month. Now I'm so picky with my brows that I won't even attempt to find someone new in Chicago; I've become a pro at doing my own. I will even trim them! My best advice is to get them groomed by a professional once a year and maintain them yourself.

THE PAINT (MAKEUP)

The amount of makeup I wear depends on where I'm going and what I'm doing, but the majority of the time, my face takes 2 minutes flat: Apply tinted moisturizer (with sunscreen), fill in my brows, and put on a little mascara. I hate doing a full face of makeup every morning, and if I'm just running around doing errands with the kids and cooking at home, then who cares? It's funny though, because I've always said I was a makeup artist in another life. I enjoy taking my time and going all out with my makeup occasionally. Since I don't apply a full face often, it's fun and exciting when I actually indulge. I even do my own makeup for events sometimes.

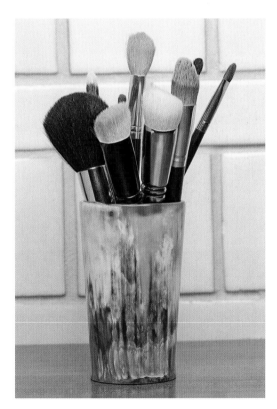

Following are a couple of techniques:

Contouring

Ya know how everyone has that one thing on their face they would fix if they could? Well, mine is the tip of my nose—it looks long from certain angles. Now look, I'm not complaining (there are worse things going on in the world than not liking my nose), but it is the one thing that sometimes drives me crazy in pictures. Years ago, there was a rumor that I got a nose job, which made me laugh considering that's the one thing I actually want done. (I would never have the surgery, though!)

Luckily, my makeup artist has made it so that I don't have to get plastic surgery to feel confident in photos. He taught me contouring. Or as I like to call it, a nose job in a brush. Contouring is glorious. But the makeup has to be applied correctly; otherwise it's easy to look like a drag queen! I don't do it on myself unless I know I'll be photographed. And I only contour a little bit. I've had makeup artists literally draw brown and white lines all over my face and blend them to make my entire face look flawless and more defined, but I just don't have the skills to replicate that. All I do myself on those special occasions is contour my nose: After you've applied foundation, put darker foundation or concealer on the outside of your nose right up the sides. Then, put a light line of concealer down the middle of your nose and blend with a sponge. I follow it up with highlighter down the center of my nose. I also put highlighter on my cheekbones after the bronzer and/or blush and in the corner of my eyes to open them up.

> My makeup artist has made it so that I don't have to get plastic surgery to feel confident in photos. He taught me contouring. Or as I like to call it, a nose job in a brush.

Fake Lashes

Applying fake individual lashes seems intimidating, but it's actually pretty easy. If I can do it, then you can too. When you have finished applying your makeup, put eyelash glue on the plastic container that the lashes come in. With tweezers, grab each lash one by one and dip the base lightly in the glue. Apply the lashes on your lash line slowly and with confidence. If you are telling yourself you can't do it, then you won't be able to. Just know that you've got this! I switch up my hand position for the right eye and grab the lash the opposite way with the tweezers. Try it a few different ways to see how you are most comfortable. Depending on where I'm going, I either just do a few on the outside or put them on the entire lash line for more drama.

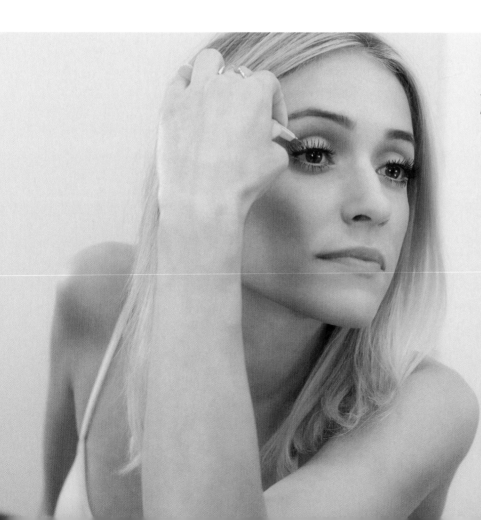

Applying individual lashes for a full look

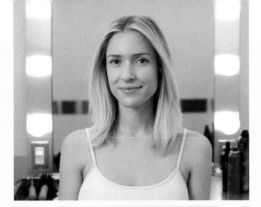

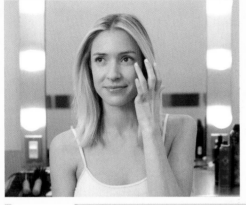

THE LOOKS

The Daytime Face

▶ Apply tinted moisturizer.

▶ Fill in brows.

▶ Put on mascara.

▶ Apply blush.

▶ Apply lightly tinted lipgloss.

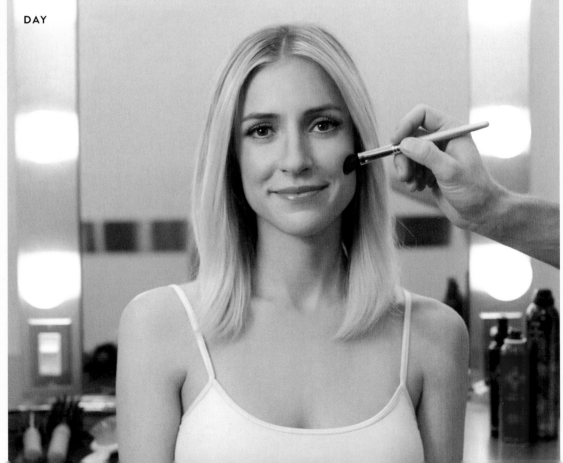

DAY

The Nighttime Face

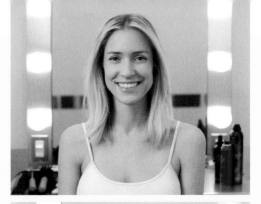

- Apply eyeshadow.
- Put brown liner on the outside lid and inside of upper lid.
- Put mascara on tip lashes.
- Apply foundation.
- Apply light powder to conceal everything.
- Brush light eyeshadow underneath eyes.
- Finish eyes with mascara on lower lashes.
- Fill in brows.
- Apply bronzer and blush.
- Add highlighter on nose, cheekbones, and inner eyes.

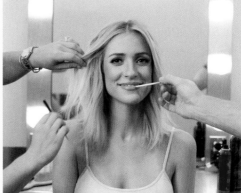

NIGHT

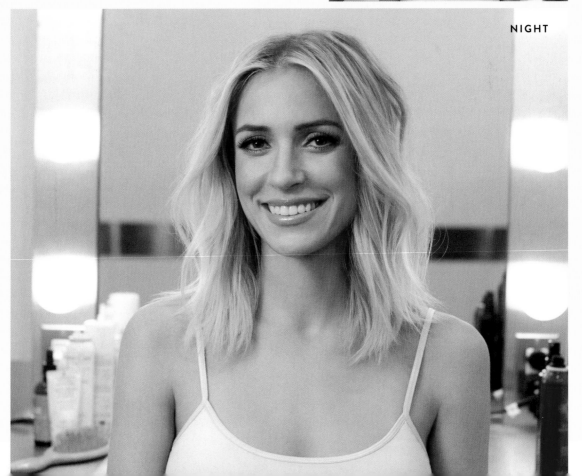

Picture Ready

If I'm doing my own makeup for an event, I tend to put on a little more makeup than I normally wear—usually a slightly darker eye, more mascara, plus fake lashes. I do everything as for the nighttime face, but I also use concealer under my eyes and contour my nose. I will usually apply brown eyeliner on the lower inside rim of my eyes as well.

Here are some of the best tips from my makeup artist, Spencer Barnes. He's a genius and works with many faces in Hollywood. He nails the glow-y, sun-kissed look but can also do dramatic, bold looks in a flash.

▶ **BRONZER** is one of the best cosmetics to warm up the face and give subtle shape and definition with a glow. Don't forget the neck and décolletage!

▶ Use a **LASH CURLER** to help your lashes extend upward. Longer-looking lashes catch attention and make your eyes appear awake.

▶ **BROWN MASCARA** on the bottom lashes as well as the top gives softer definition to the eyes. Similarly, try using a **BRONZE OR GOLDEN WATER-RESISTANT PENCIL** in the lower water line to create depth, sheen, and interest. Or try a little color for a pop—navy or smoky plums are amazing for brown eyes and warm bronzes and earthy purples are great for blue or green eyes.

▶ A **VIBRANT LIPSTICK** (creamy or velvet matte is best) can instantly take a casual look to business or day into night. You can create an alluring, confident, or playful pout depending on your mood.

▶ Makeup is a tool, not a duty or a chore, so **HAVE FUN AND DON'T BE AFRAID** to experiment. Step out of your routine sometimes to switch it up. To start, focus on just one of your features and see how different applications give you a different edge. You can use makeup to tell whatever story you want—whether fresh-faced, dramatic, or anything in between.

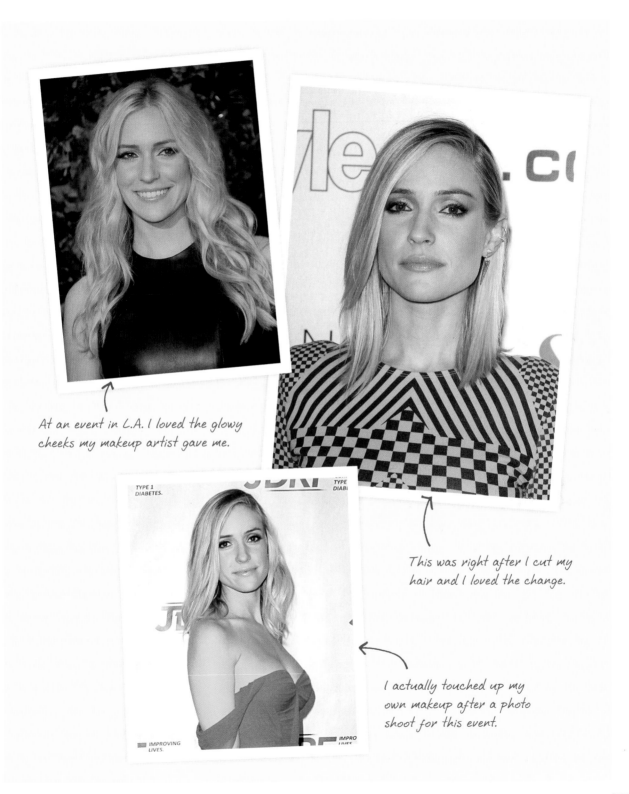

At an event in L.A. I loved the glowy cheeks my makeup artist gave me.

This was right after I cut my hair and I loved the change.

I actually touched up my own makeup after a photo shoot for this event.

Balancing It All

Beauty is being comfortable in your own skin and taking care of your body from the inside out. When I'm eating well and working out, my skin looks the best, which makes it possible to get away with minimal makeup most days. Regarding my hair, a good base haircut does wonders. I've realized that looking perfect and always being done up just isn't for me. My confidence in my physical self comes from being healthy (though a great hair day never hurts, of course!). Most days, there are a million things I'd rather be doing than following a 20-step makeup routine. Then on those days when I do take the time to get ready, I enjoy it. Either way, I believe being happy and healthy are the first steps—your glow and your natural beauty will shine through.

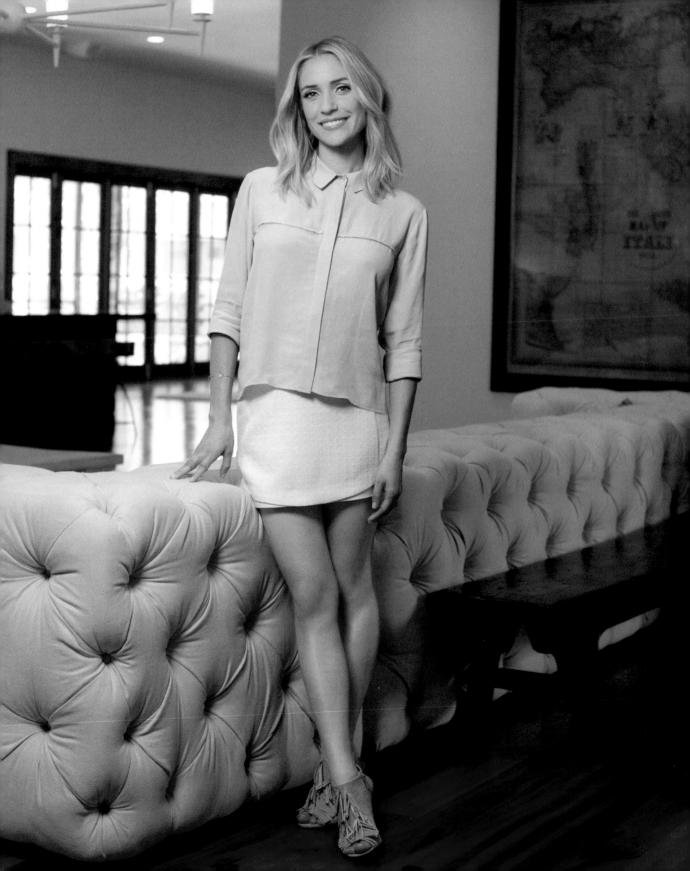

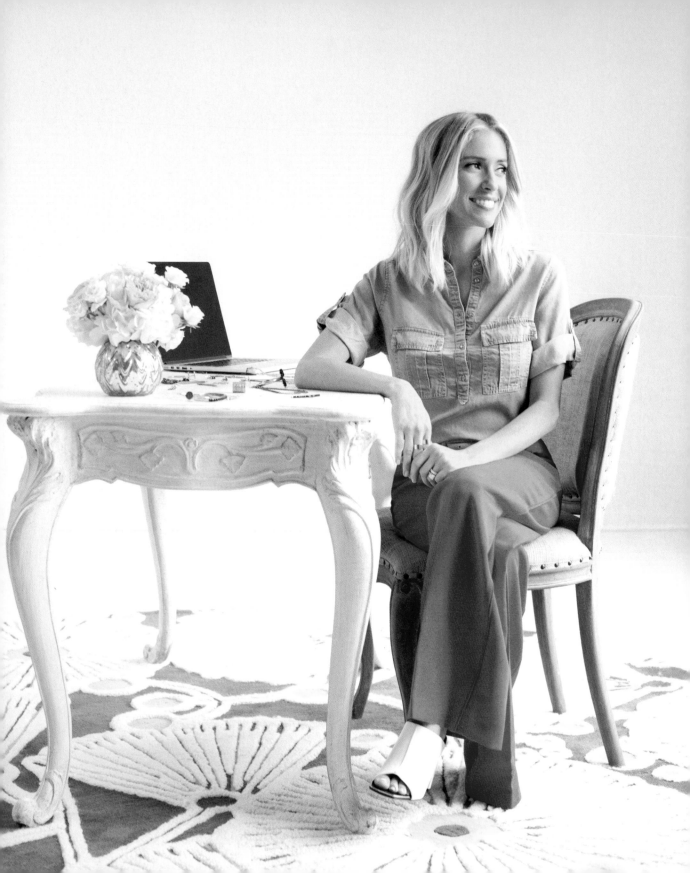

HBIC*

I'VE BEEN A WORKING GIRL SINCE I WAS 14. NOT BECAUSE I HAD TO, but because I wanted to. I loved the feeling of making my own money. Even as a kid, it gave me power and independence. I liked that it was mine and I could do what I wanted with it. Seeing different family dynamics after my parents divorced made me realize that I never wanted to rely on anyone for money, especially a man. I wanted to be able to survive on my own and not have money be a reason to be with someone. Plus, I felt bad taking money from my dad. I didn't want to owe anybody anything. I was much happier earning my own cash so I could buy what I wanted—then, clothes and candy; now, shoes and kitchen gear—without having to ask anyone else.

* Head Bitch in Charge

Besides babysitting in junior high, my first job was working at a Bikram yoga studio in Laguna Beach. My main responsibility was putting the sweaty towels in the washing machine and wiping down the mirrors in the studio. Not very glamorous! After that, at age 15, I became a hostess at a nice restaurant 2 minutes from my house. I loved that job because everyone I worked with was older and treated me like a young adult. My entire childhood, I yearned to be older. I felt like I fit in at my hostess job, plus it opened up the world to me beyond high school. I kept it up until MTV came and we started filming *Laguna Beach* my junior year of high school. Since we got paid to do the show and it took up every weekend for 9 months, that became my job.

After *Laguna Beach*, I liked the idea of being a TV host and being in front of the camera. I even wanted to study broadcast journalism at college to pursue being a host. Not long after starting at Loyola Marymount University in Los Angeles, I booked a hosting job: a show called *Get This Party Started* on UPN, where we found people affected by different tragedies, such as Hurricane Katrina, gave them the necessities they lost, and threw them a party. The show required my traveling around the country, so I dropped out of college to film the first season. After the show got canceled, everyone around me encouraged me to pursue acting, since it seemed like the normal path after reality TV and hosting. I just went with it, since I wasn't exactly sure what I wanted to do. Ultimately, I acted for about 5 years, doing five movies and a few guest spots on TV shows like *CSI: NY*. I enjoyed acting. Looking back now, I wish I had put more time and energy into it, because I didn't take it seriously then, and it showed in the work.

Around that time, *The Hills* made me an offer I couldn't refuse. Deciding to go back to reality TV was a tough decision, since I had tried so hard to get away from that genre and be taken seriously as an actress (which was funny, considering I didn't take myself seriously). Ultimately, I viewed my financial security as more important, so I accepted the offer. But one thing was different: I would look at *The Hills* strictly as a job (not as my identity) and have fun with it. I knew the character they wanted me to play, and this time, since it was my decision, playing the villain would be enjoyable. I'm incredibly thankful and happy with my decision, because it opened up many more doors for me by getting my name back out there.

DREAMS DO COME TRUE

Around age 22, not long before *The Hills* wrapped, I did some soul searching to identify what made me happy and what I loved doing. Being lucky enough to be on TV and in photo shoots, I sometimes felt like I was getting paid to play dress-up.

Through that, I started to love fashion, and of course that included shoes. Once I gained some confidence, I decided to go after what I wanted. I thought that having a shoe line could be a reality if I really wanted it and was willing to fight for it. I mean, someone gets to have that job—why not me?

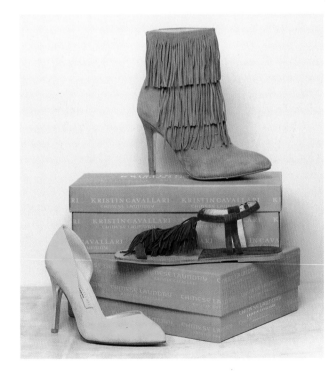

Shoes have always been a big part of my life. My first "heels" were a pair of white lace-up open-toe sandals with a little square heel. I got them in fifth grade and absolutely loved them. My mom thought I was ridiculous because I fell whenever I wore them, but I was obsessed. They made me feel like a lady. Since then, I've been a confirmed shoe girl. When I was 18, I started an inspiration book for shoes. I tore pictures of footwear I loved from magazines and printed pictures off the computer and pasted them in the book. I drew a few (horrible) sketches and even added swatches from a fabric store. That book sat in my desk drawer for years. I added ideas constantly. I imagined one day it could be inspiration for my own line. It was a pipe dream, but I didn't mind that I was living in a fantasy world.

There were a few false starts. I was vocal with my agents about wanting a shoe line, and they started setting up meetings for me. One manufacturing company wanted to produce my shoes, but I had to find a buyer (i.e., a department store). At the time, no stores would take me on because I hadn't proved myself in that world yet.

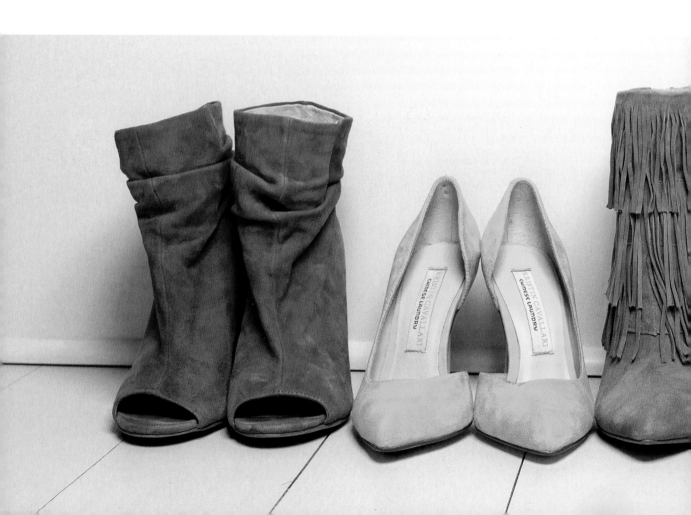

Then I met with a big shoe designer whom I loved. He was thrilled about the possibility of doing a shoe line together and asked me a million questions about the direction I wanted to take. He thought I had great ideas. I couldn't wait to get going. It was all bliss until I found out it wasn't happening. He decided to work with another celebrity (although that shoe line never saw the light of day either). I was crushed. How could it not happen after so many months of talking about it? Well, if I've learned anything in the entertainment business, it's that people blow smoke. They tell you exactly what you want to hear and then never follow up—or they go with what they think is the next best thing.

I could have easily been so discouraged that I threw in the towel at that point. And I was devastated! But I decided to keep going—I saw it as the world's way of testing me to determine how badly I wanted my shoe line. I learned from acting

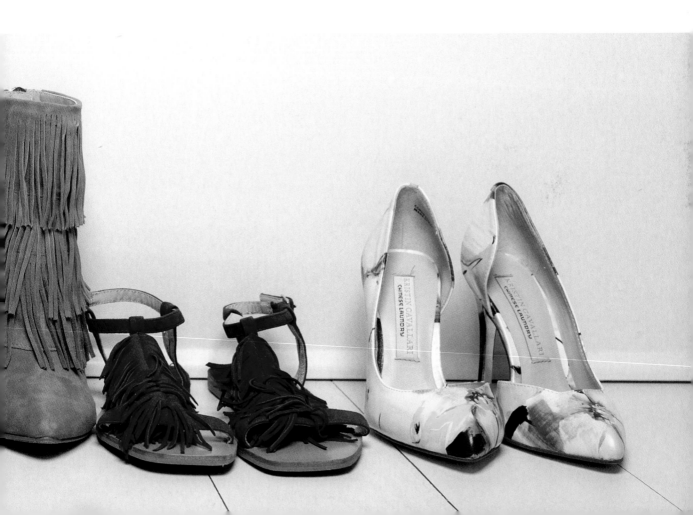

My Top Five Favorites from My Shoe Line

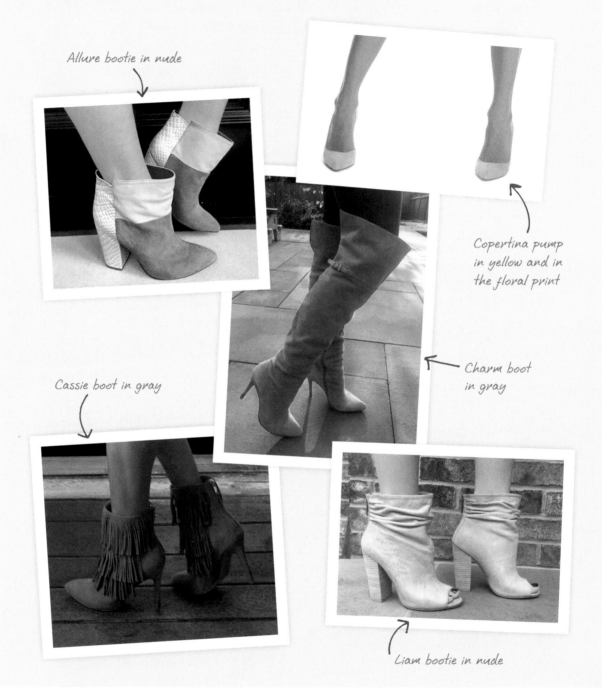

Allure bootie in nude

Copertina pump in yellow and in the floral print

Charm boot in gray

Cassie boot in gray

Liam bootie in nude

that you *will* be told no numerous times. You can't let it get you down or stop you. So I decided to use the experience with this designer as motivation and push harder. I was going to prove to him that he made a bad decision.

Approximately a year after that, I met with Chinese Laundry about writing an online fashion blog for them. I thought it was a great idea and was excited about the work, but I told them from the get-go that the main reason I was interested was the hope that our relationship could turn into my own line one day. Luckily, we loved working with each other. Not long after we started the blog, Chinese Laundry decided to make my dreams come true and give me a shoe line! I will never forget the thrill of hearing that news and then seeing my first collection come out. Plus, being told no a few times earlier made me appreciate what I had with Chinese Laundry that much more. To fight for your dreams—and have them materialize—is the best feeling in the world.

::

Shoes give women confidence and make them feel sexy. Shoes make the outfit—they are truly the best part!

::

Shoes give women confidence and make them feel sexy. Shoes make the outfit—they are truly the best part! Having my own shoe line meant I could prove that looking and feeling great doesn't have to cost a fortune. It's imperative: Everything I design is affordable. Most people can't spend $900 on Christian Louboutins—and I don't think you have to to look and feel great! My line began with classic styles that you could wear forever and mix with everything in your closet. Then I decided to expand into a trendier space as well, with some new staples. Shoes are a great way to stay on trend without having the trend overpower your overall look. I love giving women the ability to feel good about themselves and show who they are!

Working in the shoe business has been fascinating for numerous reasons. Seeing a shoe go from a sketch to a real product is an incredible feeling. And learning what goes on behind the scenes to make that happen has been an eye-opener. My heart has broken numerous times over shoe designs that I absolutely loved but never came to fruition. Buyers from the world's department stores decide if they want to carry a particular shoe, and that can make or break production of each model. I've fought and pushed for certain shoes again and again, to no avail. Buyers can also say they want to see a specific type of shoe—at one point, for example, they requested more date-night shoes. Bottom line, they are in charge. But I still have final say on what shoes we present to the buyers, so that gives me creativity and control. In other words, if I'm not happy with a particular shoe design, then it won't even get as far as the buyer. I have to believe in every shoe I put my name on, and I'm happy with every single shoe I've done. Of course, I still have my favorites!

The process of designing shoes is ongoing; I'm constantly bookmarking colors, other shoes, fabrics, and ideas that I see. The first step for each new line, about a year before it eventually comes out, begins when Chinese Laundry sends me the trend forecast, which includes themes (such as military, pop art, black and white, etc.) and the hot colors for that season. Concurrently, I've been thinking of what I want to design next, so I'll send Chinese Laundry my specific ideas and inspiration photos (including exactly what I like or don't like about a particular picture) for the upcoming season. Once they've received my inspiration, they draw sketches of our ideas, called "color ups," and send them to me for review. I tell them what I like or want to change. By now, they know my style and my preferences, so it's not often that I don't like a shoe and want to drastically change something. Sometimes there is a shoe I must have and there's no swaying me. We typically design more shoes than we'll produce, since buyers generally pass on a few models. I have to say, it's such a good feeling to love a shoe so much, push for it, and stick to my guns about every last detail, and then it ends up being one of my bestsellers. I love hearing how much girls love my shoes! When they send me pictures of the shoes via social media, it makes my day. Being able to create happiness like that is an incredible feeling.

> I love hearing how much girls love my shoes! . . . Being able to create happiness like that is an incredible feeling.

How to Be a Respected HBIC

In the entertainment business, you hear everything about everybody. If someone is always late or mean, you will hear about it. Likewise, I've heard people praise others for their kindness and positivity. That's what I want people to say when I leave the room. These are the rules I live by:

▶ Always be on time, or even a few minutes early. People who are consistently late drive me crazy! Being late is disrespectful to the other person, implying their time isn't as valuable as yours. If you are going to be late, even by 5 minutes, call and let the person know. Everyone appreciates a courtesy call.

▶ Always handwrite thank-you notes. I can't tell you how many compliments I've gotten on this. Handwritten notes are nearly a lost art, but I think they're a necessity. (Thanks for the great advice, Mom!)

▶ Surround yourself with people who inspire you, support and encourage your ideas, and bring you up. To be honest, I used to disagree with this statement, because I didn't want to believe it (I hung out with some not-so-great people at one point). But I've learned that you really are who you hang out with.

▶ Stay true to your word. If you say you are going to do something, then do it. Otherwise, don't say it at all. Broken promises are another pet peeve of mine!

▶ Focus on positives and don't dwell in the past. There are things I regret doing when I was younger, but there's nothing I can do about it now. You can only move forward. Constantly beating ourselves up is a hard way to live. Be positive.

▶ I strive to be grateful for everything I have. Looking ahead and being focused on what you want are fine, but it's important to appreciate what's already in front of you too. There's something to be said about being happy where you are, at every moment.

BRACELETS

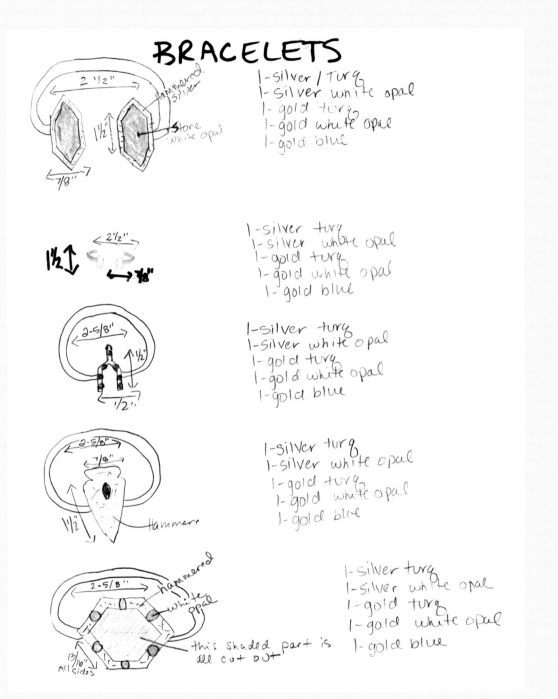

2 ½"

hammered silver

1 ½"

Stone white opal

7/8"

1 - silver / Turq
1 - silver white opal
1 - gold turq
1 - gold white opal
1 - gold blue

1 ½"   2 ½"   7/8"

1 - silver turq
1 - silver white opal
1 - gold turq
1 - gold white opal
1 - gold blue

2 - 5/8"   ½"   ½"

1 - silver turq
1 - Silver white opal
1 - gold turq
1 - gold white opal
1 - gold blue

2 - 5/8"   7/8"   1 ½"   Hammer

1 - silver turq
1 - silver white opal
1 - gold turq
1 - gold white opal
1 - gold blue

2 - 5/8"   hammered   white opal   13/16" All sides

this shaded part is all cut out

1 - silver turq
1 - silver white opal
1 - gold turq
1 - gold white opal
1 - gold blue

Sketches for Emerald Duv

BLING-BLING

After my shoe line took off, I started thinking about other areas in the accessories world that I wanted to dip my toe in. Then one of my best friends brought up the idea of partnering on a jewelry line. While I was a little nervous—since I care immensely about my girl, Chelsea, and didn't want business to hurt our friendship—I said yes.

We wanted to keep with the theme of my shoe line and make everything affordable. We wanted trendy pieces, big statement necklaces, and some smaller pieces to layer and stack with jewelry that women already own. We have different styles when it comes to jewelry. I love dainty, delicate pieces, and Chelsea is more into a boho, Malibu-beach-babe look. So we saw this collaboration as representing every girl, since it would be a great combo of both of our styles. We launched

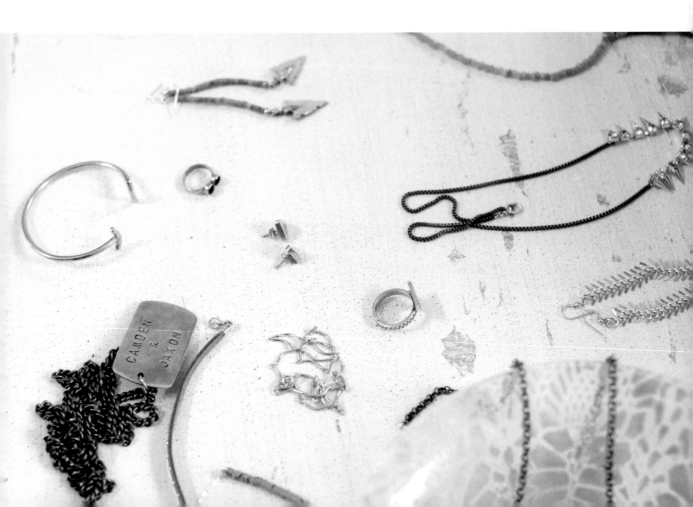

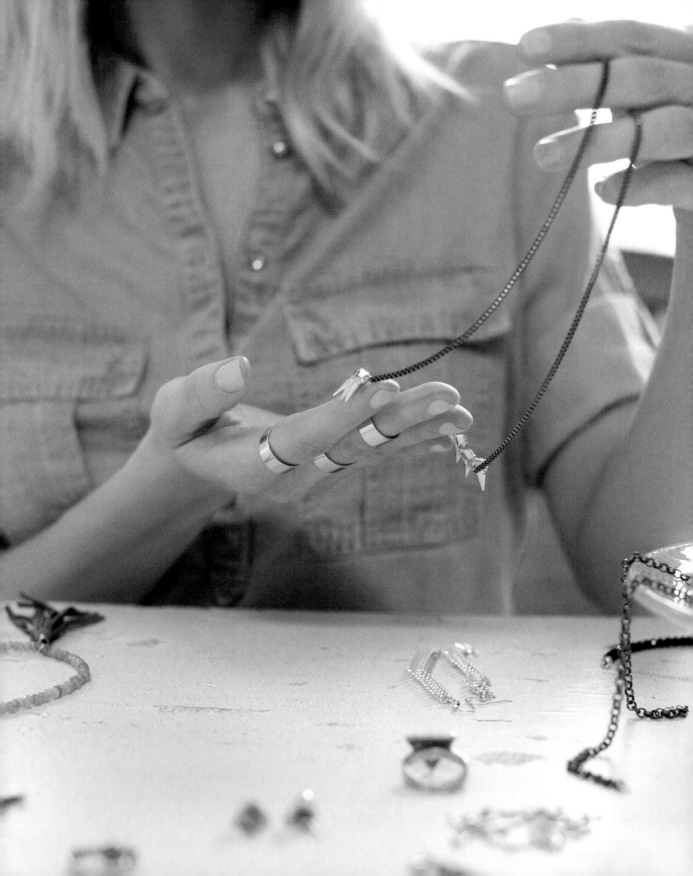

Emerald Duv in fall 2014. We came up with the name because we each have a baby with the birthstone emerald, and doves come in pairs. Since there are two of us, we thought the name made perfect sense. We changed the spelling of *dove* simply to give the name some edge.

Chelsea possesses true talent—she has been working in the jewelry world for some time and has a great eye. Our collaboration is a bit like the process of designing my shoes: I send Chelsea my ideas and inspiration, and she draws up what we both love. She sketches our ideas in pencil, a technique that has almost become a thing of the past, as most designers use computer programs these days. Chelsea knows the business well, and she has a good sense of what the buyers might want. Luckily, even if buyers don't elect to take on a certain piece, we're able to sell it on our Web site, EmeraldDuv.com. My heart doesn't have to break like it sometimes does in the shoe world! Emerald Duv has been a great collaboration. I truly enjoy creating unique jewelry for women that can make their outfit, just like shoes.

BLONDE AMBITION

Every January, I write out my goals for the coming year. It helps make the life I want come true. Creating a plan is the first step toward executing your goals. (Yep, I'm type A!) I keep it simple: usually three big goals and a few smaller ones for my career, along with a few for my family. I make sure to look back periodically throughout the year and see where everything is heading. There is no better feeling than achieving something that's on the list.

IN FRONT OF THE MIKE

Due mostly to my shoe line, I believe, doors have recently opened for me in the fashion-related hosting world, which has been incredible. My life has come full circle, since hosting is what I originally envisioned myself doing when I was 18. It's fun to be in front of the camera and talk about something as creative and exciting as fashion. Plus, hosting supports everything else I'm doing in the branding world; it keeps my name out there, and people now associate me with my shoe and jewelry lines.

Quite a lot of prep goes into hosting a TV show, especially one about fashion. When I hosted *The Fabulist* on E!, we prepped the entire week in advance. We had a game plan for each episode—we couldn't go out there and wing it. Since we talked about all of the latest trends in fashion, beauty, and lifestyle, we had to stay up-to-date and needed to identify and mention certain facts when talking about each style. I filmed the entire season when I was 7 and 8 months pregnant with Jaxon. I traveled up until my last day at 36 weeks.

Booking *The Fabulist* opened up other hosting opportunities. I will never forget the excitement of helping with the *Countdown to the 2012 Academy Awards* on *E! Live from the Red Carpet*. I was beyond nervous but also thrilled. It was an honor that E! thought of me for that! They've been great to me and have had me cohost *E! News* when I'm in L.A. I've done fill-in cohosting gigs on shows like *Access Hollywood Live* and fashion shows for Yahoo Style. *Good Morning America* has engaged me to talk about the fashion from other award shows too. The GMA segments are a funny situation: For them, I travel the night before from Chicago to New York. While the award

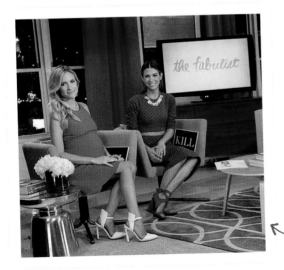

Hosting The Fabulist with Orly Shani in NYC and 8 months pregnant

show and its red carpet walk are happening live, I'm on a plane! To make it work, my publicist has to send me photos showing what everyone wore. I spend the rest of the night poring over the shots, picking out what resonates and articulating why, so I'm ready to go for the GMA call at 7:00 a.m.

THE FUTURE

One thing still on my bucket list is to produce a reality show. You can take the girl out of the reality show, but you can't take the reality out of the girl! Being behind the camera is a much less stressful place to be. I now have more control and a bigger say in what goes on and happens. Very refreshing! I've loved taking what I learned on two of the most successful reality shows to date—both the good and the bad—and applying it to my own ideas. Like with accessories, it's so satisfying to come up with the concept, develop it, and see it come to life.

Overall, producing a reality show is not too different from shoe and jewelry production. With a production company on board, we film a "sizzle reel," a short tape to pitch the show to the networks. If it sparks their interest, they'll pay for the creation of a pilot. Ideally, a pilot then screens internally, and if the execs love it, they green-light it and the pilot goes to air. I've worked really hard to get several shows to the pilot stage, but they haven't crossed the finish line. I'll admit, I've been crushed over their not making it. But, as with my shoe line, I'm not taking the no to heart too much. It's my motivation to push harder for other shows I have in the works. Stay tuned!

While my career is not entirely what I imagined it would be when I was 18, I am so lucky that I can do exactly what I am doing—which is putting my family first but still nurturing my professional side. I'm fortunate to be able to make my own hours (for the most part) and that the majority of my day is spent with my family. As long as my family is happy and healthy, everything else is cake.

Balancing It All

Moving out of Los Angeles was scary, since it was ingrained in me that to be successful in the entertainment business, you have to live in either L.A. or New York. After all, that's where almost everything happens. Professionally, I've had to make some tough choices. I had to turn down a few big hosting opportunities because they filmed every week in L.A. With my family, it would just be too hard. First of all, my babies are too young right now. I wouldn't want to be gone that much, and traveling back and forth every week would be too difficult. Also, Jay can't leave Chicago, so there's no chance for us to relocate in a better place for my career. That is a sacrifice but one I'm okay with for now. When Jay is done with football and we have more flexibility in the family schedule, it may be a different story. Then working in L.A. or even New York won't be as difficult, and acting jobs (which I still do and enjoy), more hosting, and even producing will be easier to fit in. This is another reason why I'm lucky and thankful for my shoe and jewelry lines. They keep me creative and busy, and I'm able to do them from anywhere (except for short out-of-town meetings, which I can make work).

Overall, I feel pleased with my balance. I've been able to pursue my professional dreams—from hosting, acting, and producing to designing shoes and jewelry—and have them fit within my life. Maybe it's because of my drive and my unwillingness to stop until I get what I want, or maybe it is truly just luck, but I'm blessed. I thank my lucky stars every day.

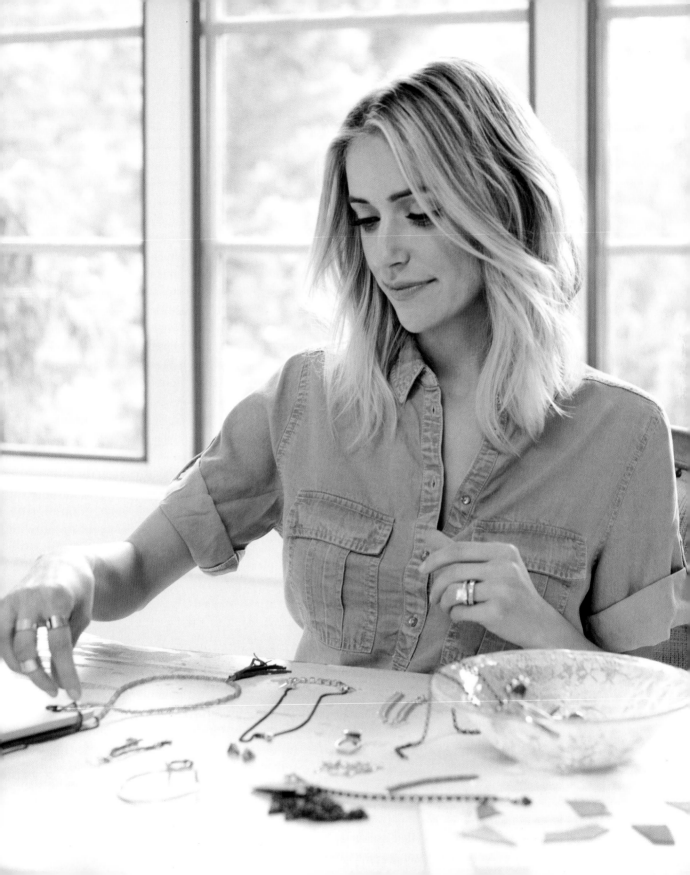

Recipes

CASHEW PANCAKES
WITH CINNAMON BROWN BUTTER

Pancakes are a favorite weekend breakfast at my house. Cashew flour adds protein and won't make your blood sugar spike. **MAKES 4 SERVINGS**

Cinnamon Brown Butter

½ cup unsalted grass-fed butter

2 teaspoons real maple syrup

¾ teaspoon ground cinnamon

¼ teaspoon fine-grain sea salt

Pancakes

1¼ cups cashew flour

1 teaspoon baking powder

½ teaspoon ground cinnamon

¼ teaspoon fine-grain sea salt

2 large eggs

½ cup coconut milk

1 tablespoon coconut oil, melted + more for cooking

2 tablespoons real maple syrup

1 teaspoon vanilla extract

1   To make the cinnamon butter: Cook the butter in a small saucepan over medium heat for 8 to 10 minutes, or until golden brown, stirring occasionally. Whisk in the maple syrup, cinnamon, and salt. Remove from the heat and set aside.

2   To make the pancakes: In a large bowl, whisk together the flour, baking powder, cinnamon, and salt. In a medium bowl, whisk together the eggs, coconut milk, 1 tablespoon coconut oil, the maple syrup, and vanilla. Add the wet ingredients to the dry and mix to combine.

3   Place a large skillet or griddle over medium heat and add a teaspoon or so of coconut oil. When the oil has melted and the pan is hot, add ¼- to ⅓-cup dollops of batter to the pan, being sure not to crowd them. Cook until bubbles appear, then flip. When browned on both sides, remove from the pan and serve immediately with the cinnamon butter drizzled on top. Add additional coconut oil as needed for cooking the next batch, and continue making pancakes until the batter is used up.

OVERNIGHT CHIA-OAT CUPS

These chia-oat cups might be the recipe I'm most excited about: They take 2 minutes to mix up; double easily; provide omega-3 fatty acids, minerals, vitamins, and soluble fiber; and overnight become a thick and creamy bowl of heaven ready for you to eat when you're running out the door the next morning.

If you have picky eaters, otherwise known as children, try these. Mine are completely addicted. Jay is a bacon-and-eggs kind of guy, and even he loves these and has asked me how to make them when I've been out of town. You can throw in whatever you want, but below are my favorite variations.

MAKES 1 SERVING

½ cup thick rolled oats

1 cup plain unsweetened almond milk

1 tablespoon chia seeds

1 teaspoon real maple syrup

In a glass container, combine the oats, almond milk, chia seeds, and maple syrup. Mix well. Cover and refrigerate overnight. In the morning, give it a good stir and enjoy.

VARIATIONS

Cinnamon Apple Delight: To the basic recipe, add 1 teaspoon ground cinnamon and half a small apple, diced.

Chocolate Almond Butter Cup: To the basic recipe, add an additional 1 teaspoon real maple syrup, 2 tablespoons almond butter, and 2 tablespoons dairy-free chocolate chips.

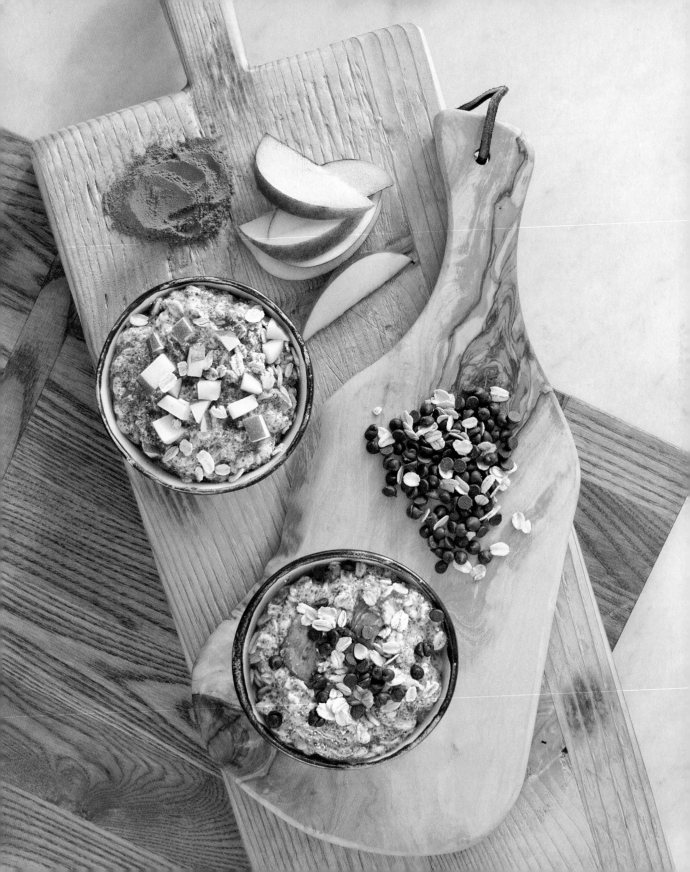

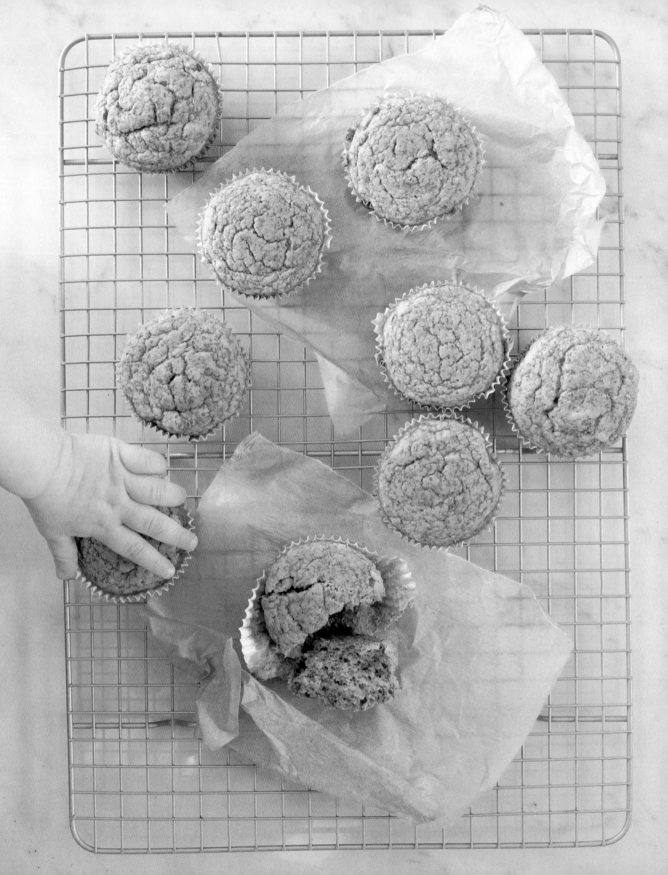

GREEN BANANA MUFFINS

Since muffins are a common snack for my family, I wanted to get some good nutrients in there with pureed spinach—success! Anytime I make these muffins, they are gone within 2 days. People might give them a funny look because of their green tint, but once they try them, no one will ask questions. Jaxon is allergic to eggs so this recipe is vegan. MAKES 18 MUFFINS

2 cups spelt flour

2 teaspoons baking powder

½ teaspoon baking soda

1 teaspoon fine-grain sea salt

1 bag (6 ounces) baby spinach (about 4 cups)

¾ cup real maple syrup

½ cup plain unsweetened almond milk

1 flax egg*

¼ cup applesauce

1½ teaspoons vanilla extract

1½ cups mashed banana (about 3 small or 2 large bananas)

1 Preheat the oven to 350°F. Line 18 muffin cups with paper liners.

2 In a large bowl, sift together the flour, baking powder, baking soda, and salt. In a food processor or blender, combine the spinach, maple syrup, almond milk, flax egg, applesauce, and vanilla and process until completely pureed. Add the wet ingredients and the banana to the dry ingredients and stir until well combined.

3 Fill each muffin cup about three-quarters full. Bake for 20 to 25 minutes, or until a toothpick inserted in the center of a muffin comes out clean. Let cool at least 10 minutes.

A flax egg is 1 tablespoon ground flaxseed plus 3 tablespoons water. Let set for about 15 minutes until it becomes a gooey consistency.

MACA TURMERIC LATTE

I don't drink coffee that often because it's acidic, so I make these maca lattes instead. Maca is a superfood that has been cultivated in the Andes of Peru for centuries. It has tons of vitamins, increases energy, is great for skin, and balances mood. **MAKES 1 SERVING**

1 cup plain unsweetened almond milk

1" fresh turmeric, grated (optional)

1 teaspoon ground turmeric

1 teaspoon maca powder

¼ teaspoon ground cinnamon

1 teaspoon real maple syrup

In a saucepan, whisk together the almond milk, fresh turmeric (if using), ground turmeric, maca powder, cinnamon, and maple syrup. Warm over medium heat until it reaches the desired temperature. Enjoy.

MOM'S PEANUT BUTTER CHICKEN

This is a favorite dish that my mom often made for my brother and me, and I'm happy to share it now with my own children. Marinate the chicken the night before, then serve with a big salad for an easy, healthy dinner.

MAKES 4–6 SERVINGS

½ cup organic peanut butter

½ cup grapeseed oil

¼ cup white wine vinegar

¼ cup tamari (see note on page 210)

Juice of 2 lemons

4 cloves garlic

1 teaspoon red-pepper flakes

1" fresh ginger, peeled and chopped

2 pounds chicken tenders

1 In a food processor, combine the peanut butter, oil, vinegar, tamari, lemon juice, garlic, red-pepper flakes, and ginger and process until fully combined. Add a few drops of water, if necessary, to reach a smooth consistency.

2 Place the chicken tenders in a resealable plastic bag or a baking dish. Pour the marinade over the chicken and use your hands to ensure it is well coated. Refrigerate and let marinate for at least 3 hours or overnight.

3 Heat a grill to 350° to 400°F or a grill pan over medium-high heat. Thread the chicken tenders onto skewers. Grill for 3 to 4 minutes on each side, or until no longer pink and the juices run clear. Remove from the skewers and serve immediately.

Note: You can also put in the oven at 350°F for 30 minutes if you don't have anyone to man the grill!

MISO SALMON

This sweet-salty glaze is so simple but so flavorful, making it the perfect match for salmon. Serve this with soba noodles and sautéed bok choy for a healthy, Asian-inspired dinner. **MAKES 2 SERVINGS**

Coconut oil, for the pan

2 wild-caught salmon fillets (6 ounces each), skin on

¼ cup Miso Glaze (page 210)

2 scallions, thinly sliced

1 Thinly coat a large skillet or grill pan with oil and heat over medium-high heat. When the pan is hot, carefully place the salmon in the pan, skin side down. Reduce the heat to medium-low.

2 Cook the salmon for about 7 minutes without moving it. It should be about three-quarters cooked and nicely browned.

3 Flip the fillets and remove the skin. Brush on the glaze. Cook for 3 to 5 minutes, or until the fish is opaque (I usually leave mine slightly raw in the middle). Remove from the heat, garnish with the scallions, and serve.

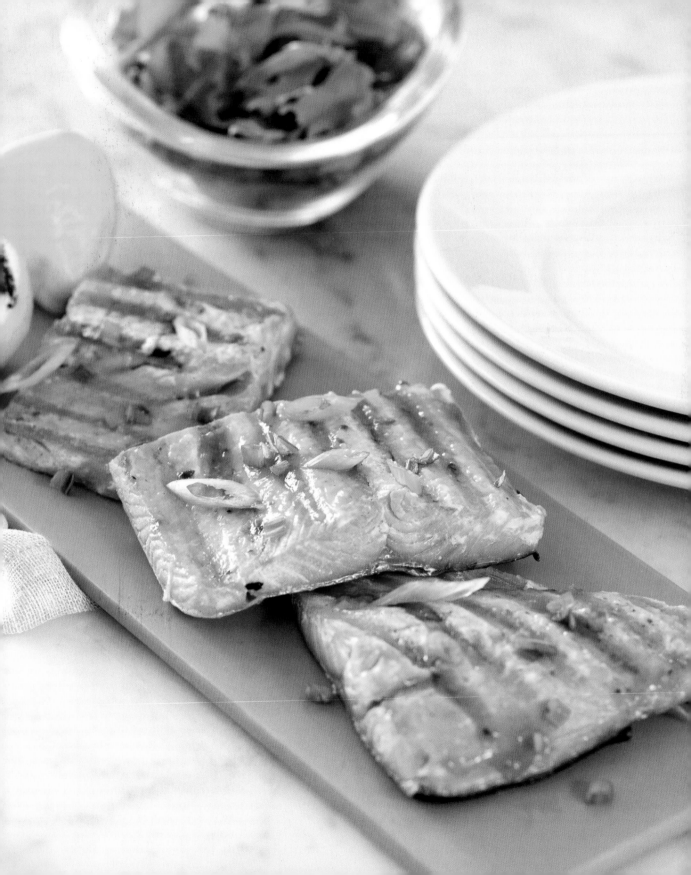

MISO GLAZE

I use this glaze for salmon and roasted Brussels sprouts, but you can use it on just about anything. It works great for grilled flank steak, grilled chicken breasts, and roasted butternut squash. It even works as a salad dressing! I like making a big batch to have on hand for spicing up weeknight dinners. **MAKES ABOUT ½ CUP**

3 tablespoons white miso paste (non-GMO)

2 tablespoons mirin*

2 tablespoons real maple syrup

2 teaspoons tamari**

1 teaspoon coconut sugar

¼ teaspoon red-pepper flakes (optional)

In a small saucepan, combine the miso, mirin, maple syrup, tamari, sugar, and red-pepper flakes (if using). Heat over medium-low heat, whisking continuously, for 2 to 3 minutes, or until the glaze begins to bubble and thickens slightly. Remove from the heat. Use immediately or store in a jar and refrigerate up to 1 week.

* Mirin is a Japanese rice wine used in cooking, similar to sake but with a lower alcohol content. Find it in the store near other Asian condiments.

** Tamari is a special Japanese soy sauce, similar to regular soy sauce, but it's usually wheat free (always read labels!). Soy sauce is a fine replacement if you can't find it. Tamari is less salty than soy sauce and a little thicker.

SLOW-ROASTED CHICKEN
WITH CHIPOTLE SAUCE

This was one of the first dishes I made when I started to cook. It's so easy that it's almost impossible to mess up. It takes only a few minutes in the morning (or the night before) and tastes like you slaved away all day. I made this one girls' night with my mom, aunt, and cousins in the first few months of my cooking, and they couldn't stop raving about it. Everyone wanted to know exactly how I prepared it, and they were shocked at how simple the recipe was. They still talk about that dinner to this day. If you aren't a fan of spicy food, omit the hot peppers. The dish will be just as good. **MAKES 4 SERVINGS**

1 medium onion, finely chopped

2 carrots, peeled and finely chopped

4 cloves garlic, peeled

2 canned chipotle peppers in adobo sauce

2 tablespoons tomato paste

1 teaspoon smoked paprika

½ teaspoon ground cumin

½ teaspoon ground turmeric

½ teaspoon pink Himalayan salt or sea salt

1 Preheat the oven to 200°F.

2 In a large roasting pan or ovenproof Dutch oven, place the onion, carrots, garlic, chipotle peppers, and tomato paste. Add about a cup of water, enough to cover the bottom of the pan, and stir until the paste dissolves.

3 In a small bowl, combine the paprika, cumin, turmeric, salt, and black pepper.

4 If needed, remove and discard any giblets or gizzards from your chicken. Use your hands to spread the spice mixture under the skin of the chicken, into all the creases and crevices. Use whatever mixture is left to rub on the outside of the skin, all over the breast and legs. Place the chicken on top of the vegetables. Pour the coconut oil over the top of the chicken and spread evenly over the skin. Cover the pan.

(continues)

¼ teaspoon ground black pepper

3–4-pound whole chicken

2–3 tablespoons coconut oil, melted

5 Roast for 9 to 9½ hours, or until a thermometer inserted in a breast registers 180°F and the juices run clear. Occasionally check the vegetables; if it looks like they may start to burn, simply add more water to the pan. When the chicken is cooked through, turn on the broiler. Broil the chicken for 7 to 10 minutes, or until the skin turns golden and crispy.

6 Remove the chicken from the pan and set aside. Carefully pour all of the veggies and liquid in the pan into a blender. Puree on high until well blended. The sauce should be the consistency of hummus. If it's too thick, add a couple of tablespoons water at a time until the desired consistency is achieved.

7 Carve the chicken and serve pieces on top of the chipotle sauce, then dig in!

DAIRY-FREE MUSHROOM-PEA RISOTTO

Creamy, delicious risotto without all the dairy. It sounds too good to be true, but it's not. Nutritional yeast is a nondairy eater's secret weapon because it adds a silky richness and slightly cheesy flavor. My mouth is already watering!

MAKES 4 SERVINGS

1 quart vegetable broth

2 tablespoons vegan butter

2 tablespoons olive oil

8 ounces cremini mushrooms, cleaned and finely chopped

2 tablespoons minced shallots

2 cloves garlic, minced

¾ cup arborio rice

¼ cup dry white wine

½ cup frozen green peas

¼ cup nutritional yeast

Pink Himalayan salt

Ground black pepper

2 tablespoons chopped chives

1 Pour the broth into a small pot. Cover, bring to a boil, and then reduce to a simmer. Keep at a low simmer while making the risotto.

2 Heat a large skillet over medium-high heat. Melt the butter and oil together. Add the mushrooms and shallots and cook for about 7 minutes, or until soft. Add the garlic and cook for another minute. Add the rice, stir well, and let it toast for a couple of minutes, until it smells nutty and starts to absorb some of the liquid in the pan. Add the white wine and stir well. Cook for about 2 minutes, or until the wine is absorbed and the pan is almost dry.

3 Reduce the heat to medium-low. Add 1 cup of the simmering broth to the rice and use a spoon to vigorously combine with the rice. Once the rice has absorbed the broth and the pan is almost dry again, add ½ cup of the broth. Stir vigorously again. Continue this process until you've used the remaining broth and the rice is tender, 20 to 30 minutes.

4 Remove from the heat. Add the frozen peas and nutritional yeast. Add salt and pepper to taste. Stir well. The heat from the risotto will warm the peas. Garnish with the chives and serve immediately.

SWEET MISO BRUSSELS SPROUTS

These Brussels sprouts are highly addictive! My favorite Miso Glaze provides a sweet-salty balance that makes these veggies irresistible. **MAKES 4 SERVINGS**

1–1¼ pounds Brussels sprouts

2 tablespoons olive oil

2 tablespoons balsamic vinegar

1 teaspoon garlic powder

2 tablespoons Miso Glaze (page 210)

1 Preheat the oven to 375°F.

2 Trim the ends off the Brussels sprouts and cut them in half lengthwise. Use your fingers to loosen the leaves so that they are less bunched together (this makes the leaves crisp up better). Place the fluffed halves into a baking dish. Add the oil, vinegar, and garlic powder. Toss so all the Brussels sprouts are coated evenly. Spread into a single layer.

3 Cover and bake for 30 minutes. Remove the cover, increase the temperature to 425°F, and bake for 10 minutes, until the leaves are crispy and brown. Remove from the oven, add the Miso Glaze, and toss to combine. Serve warm.

CHERRY-PISTACHIO QUINOA

*Quinoa provides the backdrop for crunchy pistachios and sweet cherries.
This is a great side dish for any occasion: easy to make ahead of time and
easy to double the batch. Plus, leftovers make for a healthy lunch the next day.*

MAKES 4 SERVINGS

2 teaspoons +
2 tablespoons olive oil

1½ tablespoons finely chopped shallots

1¾ cups raw quinoa, rinsed

½ cup dried tart Bing cherries, chopped

⅓ cup dry white wine

2 cups water

2–3 teaspoons lemon peel (1 lemon)

3 tablespoons lemon juice (1 lemon)

1 teaspoon fine-grain sea salt

¼ teaspoon ground black pepper

½ cup shelled pistachios, chopped

1 In a medium pot over medium heat, warm 2 teaspoons of the oil. Add the shallots and cook, covered, for about 5 minutes, or until translucent. Add the quinoa and toast it with the shallots for 2 minutes. Add the cherries, wine, and water. Cover, bring to a boil, and then reduce to a simmer. Cook for 10 to 12 minutes, or until the quinoa is tender.

2 Meanwhile, in a large bowl, whisk together the 2 tablespoons oil, the lemon peel, lemon juice, salt, and pepper until thoroughly combined.

3 When the quinoa is tender, remove from the heat, fluff with a fork, and let sit for a couple of minutes. Add the quinoa and pistachios to the bowl with the dressing. Gently toss to combine. Serve warm or slightly chilled.

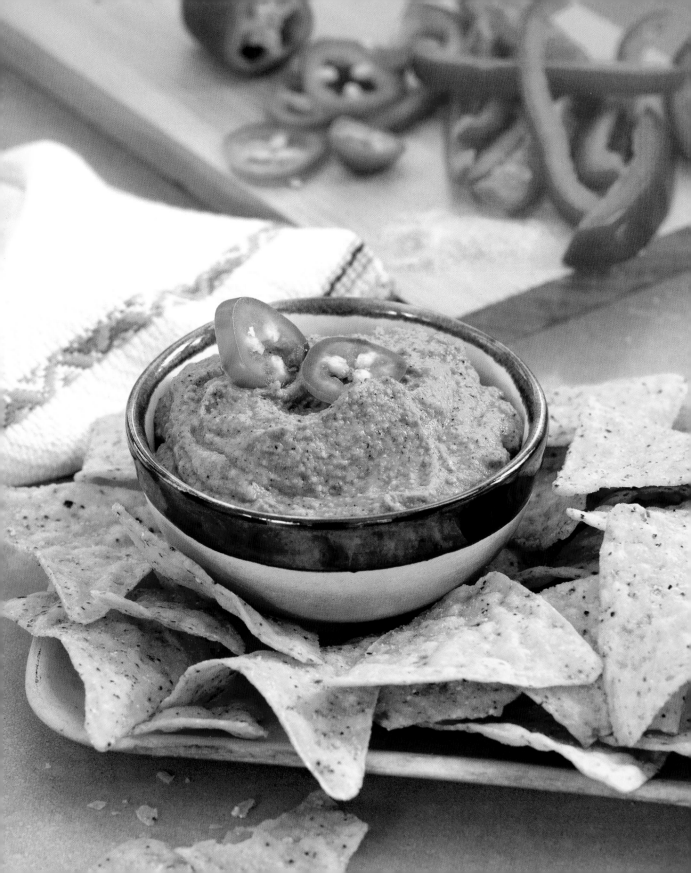

CHEESELESS QUESO DIP

Queso made from cashews? You better believe it! Don't tell anyone there isn't actual cheese in this (unless your guests have nut allergies!). They will never know. Soaked raw cashews makes the dip thick and creamy like regular queso— it's the ultimate crowd-pleaser. **MAKES 8 SERVINGS AS AN APPETIZER**

1 cup raw cashews

1 tablespoon olive oil

1 red bell pepper, seeded and finely chopped

1 small yellow onion, finely chopped

1 jalapeño chile pepper, seeded and finely chopped, wear plastic gloves when handling

2 teaspoons ground cumin

2 tablespoons chili powder

2 teaspoons minced garlic

2 cups vegetable broth

2 tablespoons white miso paste

2 teaspoons arrowroot powder or GMO-free cornstarch or tapioca powder

3 tablespoons nutritional yeast

½ teaspoon fine-grain sea salt

Tortilla chips (non-GMO), for serving

1 Place the cashews in a bowl and cover with water. Let soak for at least 8 hours or overnight.

2 Heat the oil in a medium pot over medium heat. Add the bell pepper, onion, jalapeño pepper, cumin, and chili powder. Cook over medium heat, stirring occasionally, for about 7 minutes, or until the onion is soft and the chili powder is aromatic. Add the garlic and cook for another minute. Remove from the heat and let cool slightly.

3 Meanwhile, drain and rinse the soaked cashews. Place into a food processor with the broth, miso, and arrowroot powder. Puree on high until very smooth, up to 10 minutes. Add the slightly cooled pepper mixture, nutritional yeast, and salt. Puree on high until smooth and creamy.

4 Pour the queso back into the pot used for cooking the pepper mixture. Gently bring to a simmer over low heat. Cook, whisking continuously, for about 15 minutes, or until thick and bubbly. Season to taste with additional salt. Serve immediately with the tortilla chips.

CAULIFLOWER "POTATO" SALAD

When I first made this for Jay, he said, "After having this, why would anyone make regular potato salad again?" I guess he liked it! Cauliflower is great because the taste is mild, like potatoes, but it has many more health benefits.

MAKES 6 SERVINGS

1 head cauliflower, broken into florets

5 eggs, hard-cooked and finely chopped

3 ribs celery, finely chopped

½ yellow bell pepper, finely chopped

½ orange bell pepper, finely chopped

2 tablespoons finely chopped red onions

3 large dill pickles, chopped

¾ cup mayonnaise

1 tablespoon dried dill

½ teaspoon minced garlic

½ teaspoon yellow mustard

In a large pot with a steamer basket and 3" boiling water, add the cauliflower, cover, and steam for 5 minutes, or until just tender. Let cool. Place in a bowl. Add the eggs, celery, bell peppers, onions, pickles, mayonnaise, dill, garlic, and mustard. Mix. Refrigerate until chilled.

RANCH DRESSING

This dressing is a great vegan take on a classic favorite. Make a big batch to have on hand for salads or dipping veggies. **MAKES ALMOST 2 CUPS**

1½ cups vegan mayonnaise (see Note)

¼ cup plain unsweetened almond milk

1 tablespoon apple cider vinegar

1 tablespoon fresh chopped parsley

1½ teaspoons onion powder

1 teaspoon garlic powder

½ teaspoon dried dill

¼ teaspoon ground black pepper

In a blender, combine the mayonnaise, almond milk, vinegar, parsley, onion powder, garlic powder, dill, and pepper and puree until creamy. Keep refrigerated for up to 10 days.

Note: I created this recipe while breastfeeding Jaxon, so I've only ever made it with vegan mayo, but regular mayo would work too for a nonvegan version.

BROCCOLI SALAD
WITH AVOCADO MAYO

This salad was inspired by my friend and health guru, Sarah Moore, in Nashville. I could bathe in this avocado mayo, it's so freakin' good! Just remember to soak your cashews ahead of time. **MAKES 2 SERVINGS (OR 1 FOR A BIG APPETITE!)**

¼ cup cashews

2 avocados, peeled and pitted

3 tablespoons rice vinegar

¼ teaspoon garlic powder

½ teaspoon sea salt

1 head broccoli, broken into florets

¼ cup goji berries

1 Place the cashews in a bowl and cover with water. Let soak for at least 4 hours.

2 Drain and rinse the cashews. Add to a blender with the avocados, vinegar, garlic powder, and salt and blend until smooth.

3 In a large pot with a steamer basket and 3" boiling water, add the broccoli, cover, and steam for about 5 minutes, or until just slightly soft. Let cool. Place the broccoli and goji berries in a bowl and toss with the avocado mayo. Serve immediately.

"CARAMEL" BITES

These three simple ingredients totally curb any salty-sweet cravings I have. It's amazing how similar to caramel they truly taste. I call for pink Himalayan salt because it's better for you and because its flavor is not as strong as conventional iodized salt or Celtic sea salt. **MAKES ABOUT 10 BITES**

1 cup pitted dates

Big pinch of pink Himalayan salt

Coarse sea salt

In a food processor, combine the dates and the Himalayan salt for about 30 seconds, or until a sticky ball is formed. Roll into 1 big ball, wrap in plastic wrap, and place in the freezer for 10 to 15 minutes to harden slightly. Once chilled, take out and roll into about 10 small balls. Sprinkle each with a little coarse sea salt. Store in an airtight container for up to 5 days.

OAT BALLS

These are great for a quick, easy snack. Kids love noshing on the individual balls, but you can also place the batch in a big bowl to eat with a spoon like granola.

MAKES ABOUT 15 OAT BALLS

1 cup rolled oats

½ cup almond butter

⅔ cup coconut flakes

2 tablespoons real maple syrup

½ cup chia seeds

2 tablespoons cacao nibs

2 tablespoons coconut oil, melted

⅛ teaspoon fine-grain sea salt

In a large bowl, mix the oats, almond butter, coconut, maple syrup, chia seeds, cacao, oil, and salt with your hands. Chill for 30 minutes, then roll into balls. Store in an airtight container in the fridge for up to 1 week.

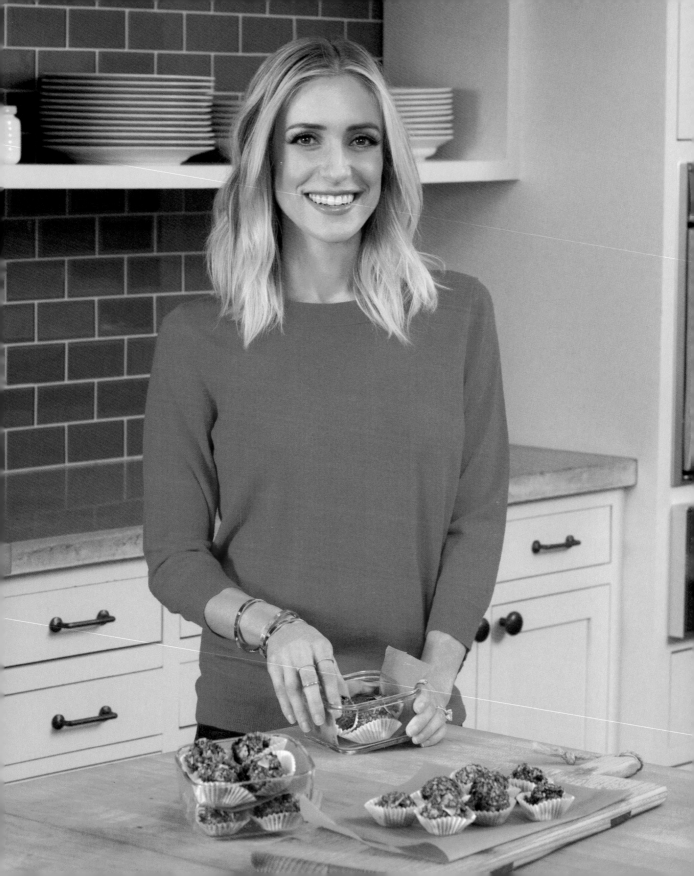

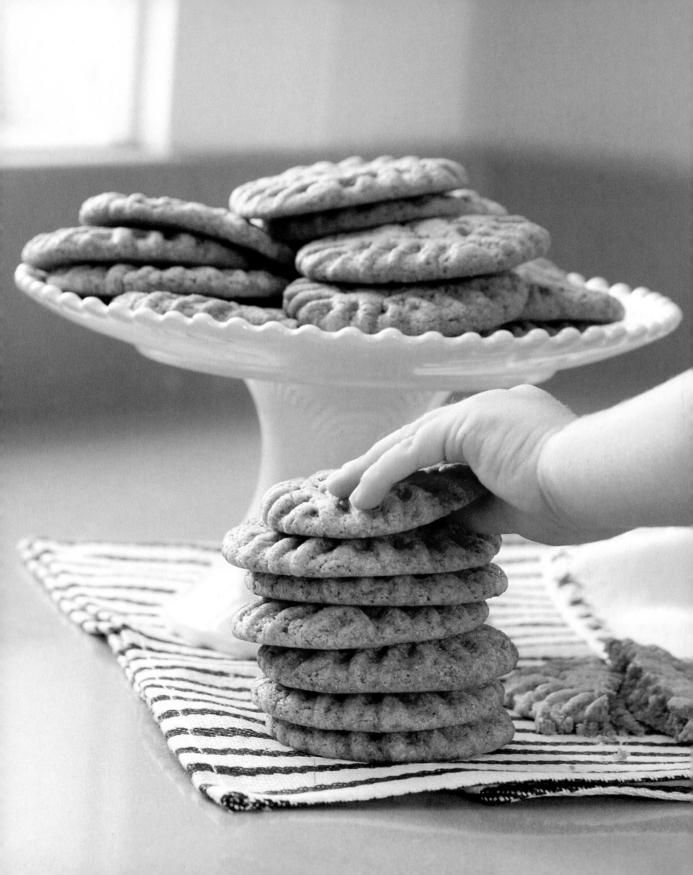

ALMOND BUTTER SUGAR COOKIES

I almost always have a cookie or some type of sweet around the house. I love these cookies so much that when I travel, I take three or four with me for the plane!

MAKES 24 COOKIES

1 stick unsalted grass-fed butter, softened

1 cup coconut sugar

½ cup almond butter

1 large egg

1½ cups oat flour

¾ teaspoon baking soda

½ teaspoon pink Himalayan salt

1 Preheat the oven to 350°F. Line 2 baking sheets with parchment paper.

2 Using a handheld or stand mixer, cream together the butter, sugar, and almond butter until fluffy. Add the egg and mix to combine.

3 In a separate bowl, mix the flour, baking soda, and salt with a spoon. Add the dry ingredients to the wet ingredients and mix well. Spoon tablespoon-size balls onto the prepared baking sheets, keeping a little distance between each ball. Bake for 10 minutes, or until they start to turn golden brown. The cookies are thin, so keep a close eye on them so they don't burn.

CHOCOLATE HEMP PUDDING

This dessert is perfect for my chocolate-loving sweet tooth. There's quite a bit of sugar in it, so don't think it's completely guilt free! It's not nearly as bad as regular pudding, though. **MAKES 4 SERVINGS**

1½ cups hemp seeds

1 cup coconut sugar

½ cup plain unsweetened almond milk

½ cup coconut water

½ cup cocoa powder

Pinch of pink Himalayan salt

2 tablespoons cacao nibs

In a powerful blender or food processor, combine the hemp seeds, sugar, almond milk, coconut water, cocoa powder, salt, and cacao until smooth. Pour into individual cups or one big bowl and refrigerate for at least 1 hour.

CHOCOLATE PEANUT BUTTER CHUNK "ICE CREAM"

Not being able to eat cow's milk means no more ice cream, but there is nothing I love more in this world. Words cannot describe how excited I am about discovering this frozen dessert made from cashews! Soaked cashews create a rich, creamy base, making them the perfect foundation for any flavor. Chocolate peanut butter is Jay's favorite flavor. **MAKES ABOUT 1 PINT**

2 cups raw cashews

1½ cups water

½ cup real maple syrup

¼ teaspoon fine-grain sea salt

¼ cup organic peanut butter

¼ cup dairy-free dark chocolate chips

1 Place the cashews in a bowl and cover with water. Let soak for at least 8 hours or overnight.

2 Drain and rinse the cashews. Place in a blender with the water, maple syrup, and salt. Puree until smooth and creamy. This is the ice-cream base.

3 Place the ice-cream base in an ice-cream mixer and mix for at least 20 minutes, until it is cold and creamy and resembles actual ice cream. Use your fingers to break the peanut butter into small, bite-size chunks. Add the chunks and the chocolate chips to the ice-cream base. Mix well to combine. Enjoy right away or tightly cover and freeze for up to 2 weeks, although it never lasts longer than a couple of days in my house!

MINT CHOCOLATE CHIP "ICE CREAM"

Mint chocolate chip has been my favorite ice-cream flavor since I was a kid. I love it so much that when I was younger, I would save part of my mint chip Blizzard from Dairy Queen and eat it for breakfast the following morning. Let's not even discuss how bad that was for me!

Even these days, were it not for my dairy intolerance, I could eat ice cream any time of day—breakfast, lunch, dinner, you name it. Now with this recipe, if I really wanted to, I could indulge for breakfast and not feel guilty.

MAKES ABOUT 1 PINT

2 cups raw cashews

1½ cups water

½ cup real maple syrup

1 tablespoon peppermint extract

¼ teaspoon fine-grain sea salt

½ cup dairy-free mini chocolate chips

1 Place the cashews in a bowl and cover with water. Let soak for at least 8 hours or overnight.

2 Drain and rinse the cashews. Place in a blender with the water, maple syrup, peppermint extract, and salt. Puree until smooth and creamy. This is the ice-cream base.

3 Place the ice-cream base in an ice-cream mixer and mix for at least 20 minutes, until it is cold and creamy and resembles actual ice cream. Stir in the chocolate chips. Enjoy right away or tightly cover and freeze for up to 2 weeks.

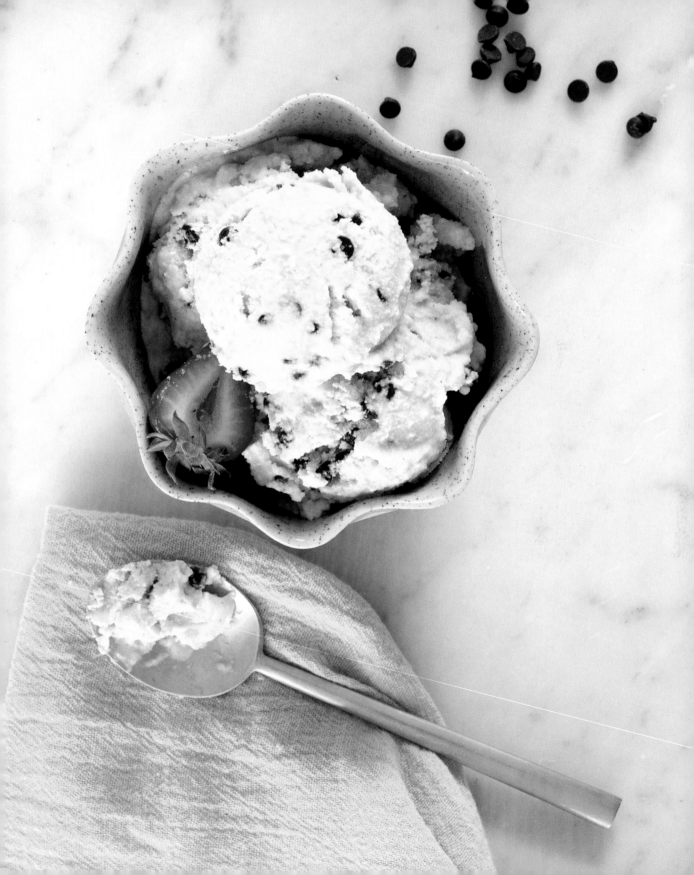

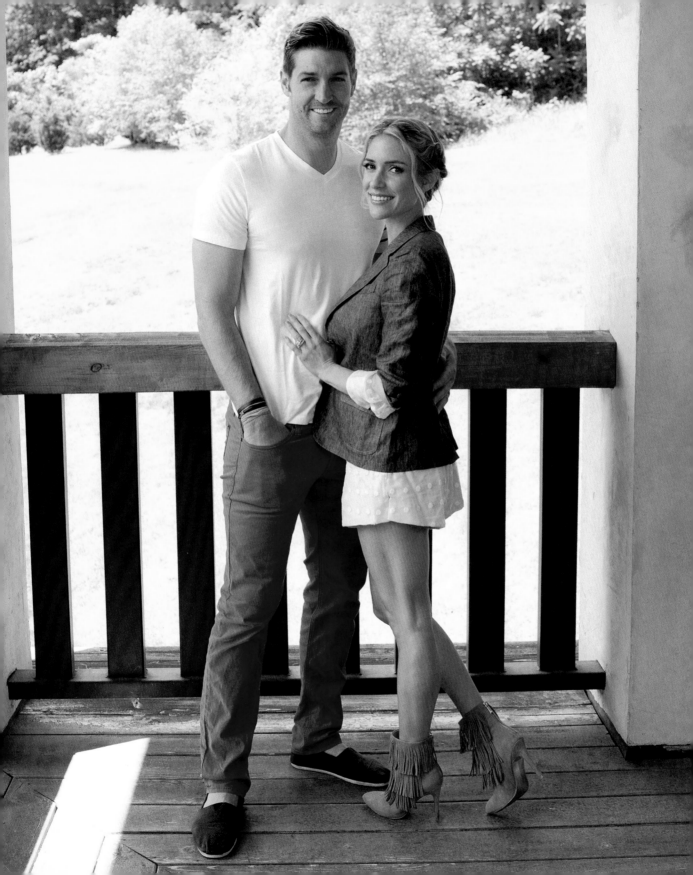

ACKNOWLEDGMENTS

I poured my heart and soul into this book and wouldn't have been able to do that without the help of many people along the way. First, I want to thank my mom and dad for instilling their wisdom and priceless life lessons in me. Dad, you have always encouraged me to go after whatever I want in life and pushed me to live up to my full potential. Your work ethic is something I am so grateful to have inherited. Mom, you have always been my biggest supporter. You taught me to believe in myself and how to love.

To my husband and children, you are the reason I exist. Jay, you have been paramount to my becoming the woman I am. You push me to be the best version of myself while keeping me grounded. My babies, Cam, Jax, and Saylor: You are my whole world, and I became me when I had you. Everything I do, I do for you.

Ellie Hutton, thank you for listening to me spill my heart out for hours and hours before I started writing and for the thoughtful, constructive criticism throughout the whole process.

Dr. Moltz, thank you for letting me spend countless hours in your office simply because I'm as obsessed with health as you are. You were an amazing sounding board, and I am so grateful to you for instilling some of your knowledge in me.

My trainer, Michael Sorrentino, I know women will appreciate your tips and workouts as much as I do.

Everyone involved in the photo shoots was a pro. To the glam squad—Scotty, Spencer, and Nicolas: Scotty, thank you for the never-ending laughter and the gorgeous hair. Spencer, you are by far one of the kindest spirits I have ever met, and I thank you for bringing your peaceful, calming energy to every set we've ever been on. Nicolas, thank you for working around my preggers belly and always bringing a smile wherever you go. Tec, this book wouldn't have turned out half as good without you—thank you for capturing precious moments with my family and for the beautiful pictures. Mary Carter, thank you for making my recipes look 10 times better than I ever could!

Susan, I can't say enough. Without your dedication, intelligence, and take-no-shit mentality, I wouldn't be where I am today. Thank you for always having my back and being the strong, assertive woman on my team. Jack, we've been through a lot together in the last 10-plus years, including lots of laughs and fun times. You go above and beyond, and it's greatly appreciated.

Mary Jo, I'm grateful for your encouragment to be my highest self.

My girls—you know who you are—I would be lost without you guys.

Everyone at the Rodale team, thank you for giving me the opportunity to tell my story and enthusiastically believing in me from the moment I stepped foot in your door.

The fans, especially the ones who have been with me since day 1: You guys have grown with me and always had my back. I've said I have the best fans in the game, and I truly mean that. Thank you for giving me a reason to keep going.

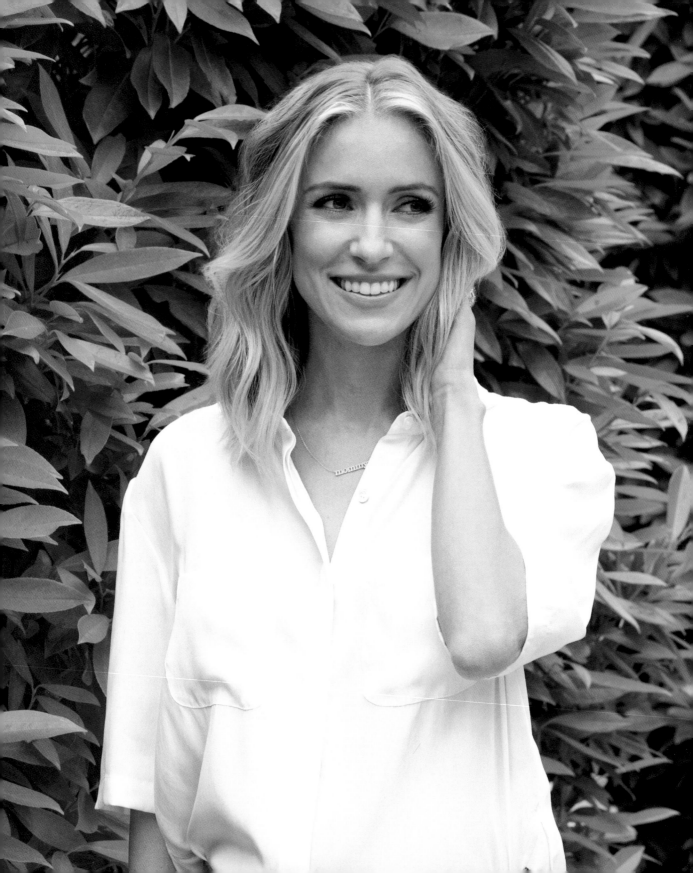

INDEX

Underscored page references indicate sidebars and tables. **Boldface** references indicate photographs.

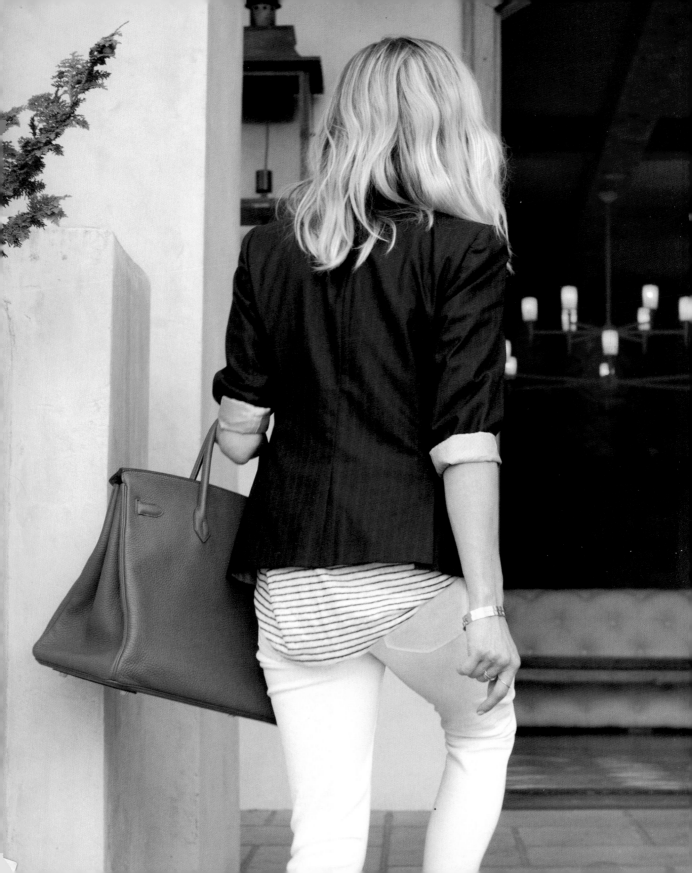